Hypothyroidism - New Aspects of an Old Disease

Edited by Ifigenia Kostoglou-Athanassiou

Published in London, United Kingdom

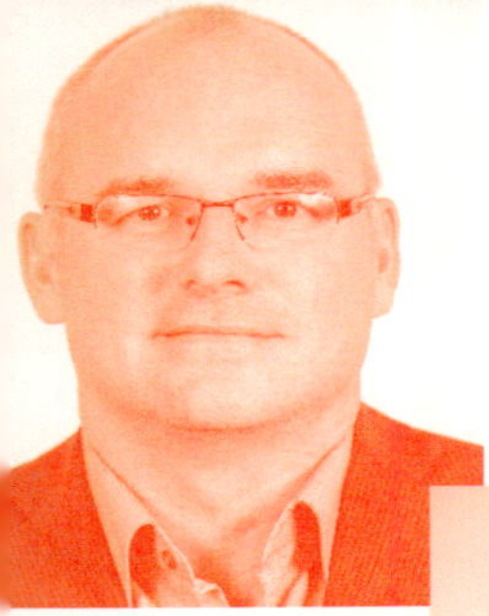
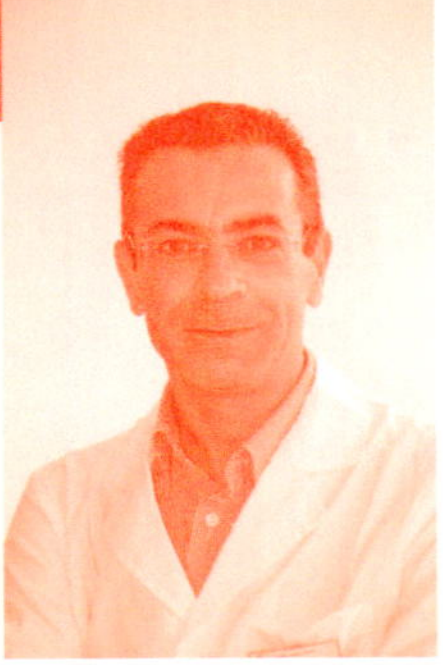
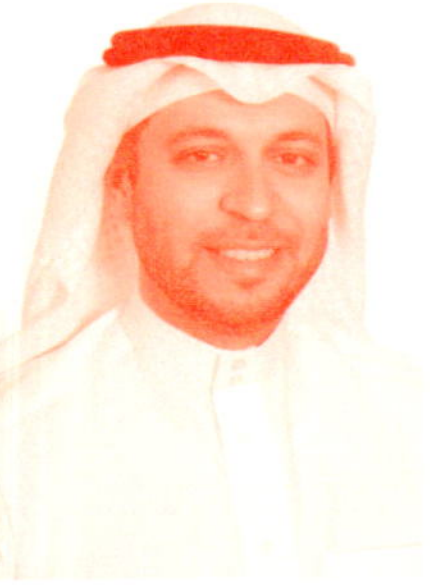
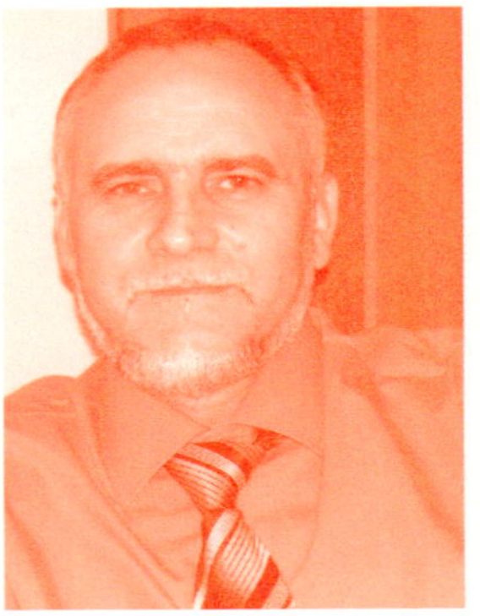
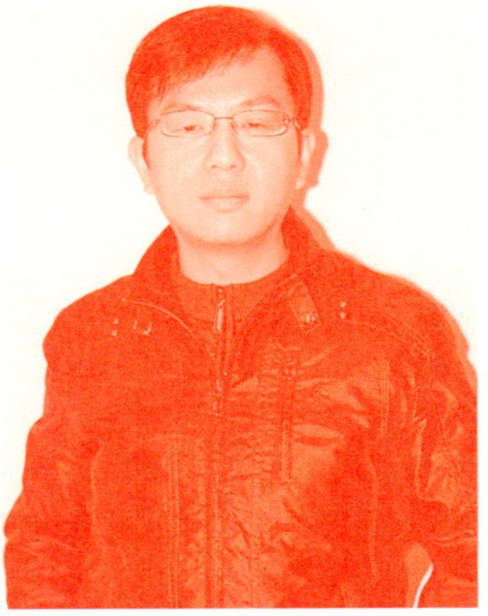
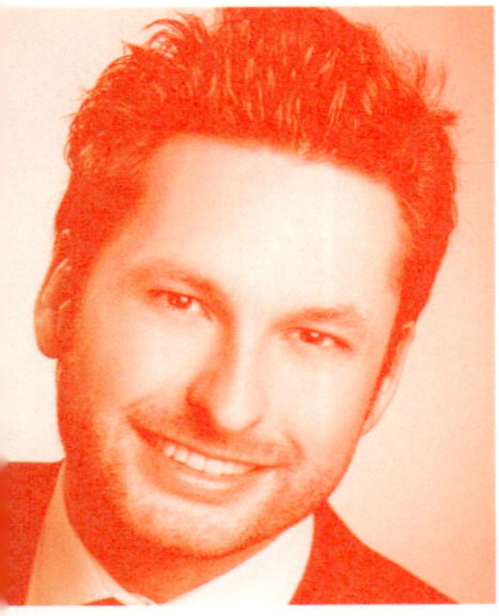
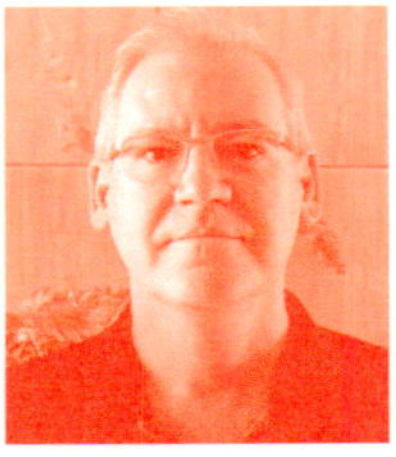

IntechOpen

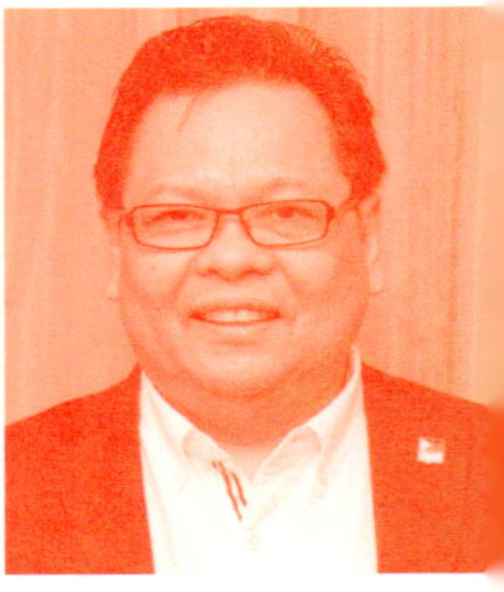
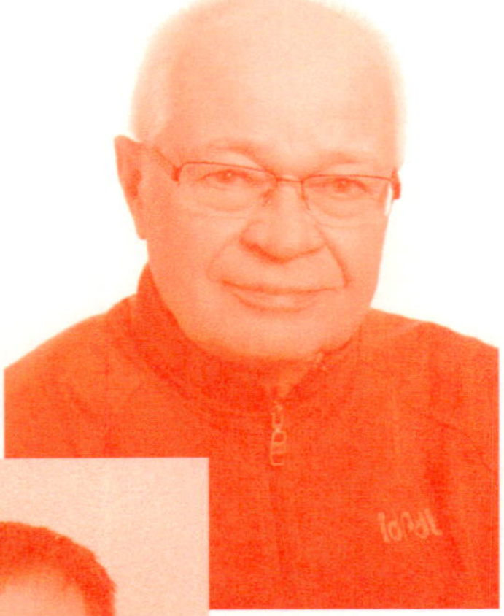
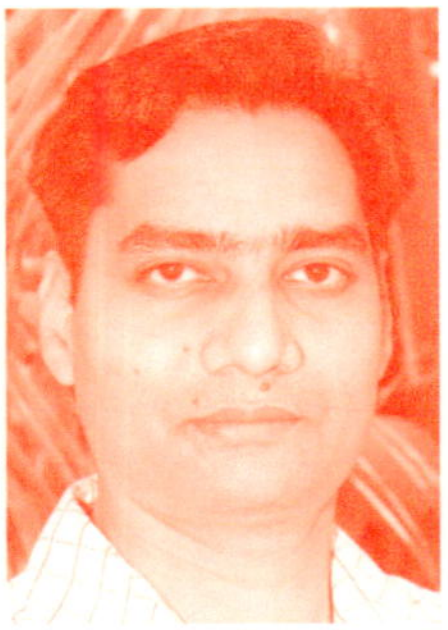
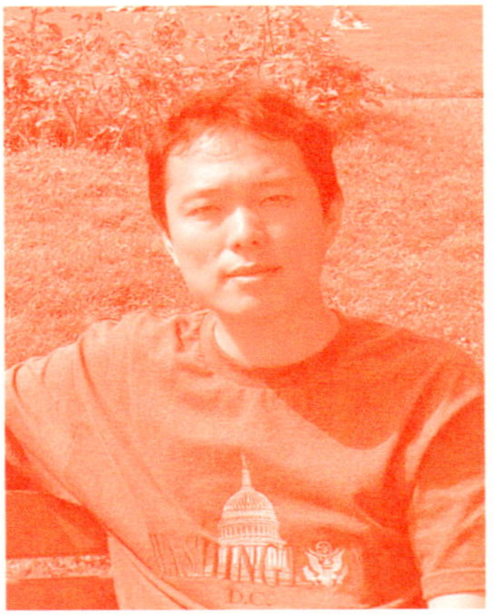
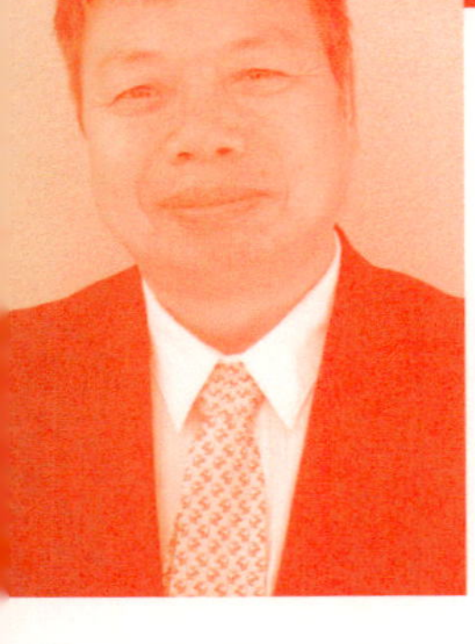
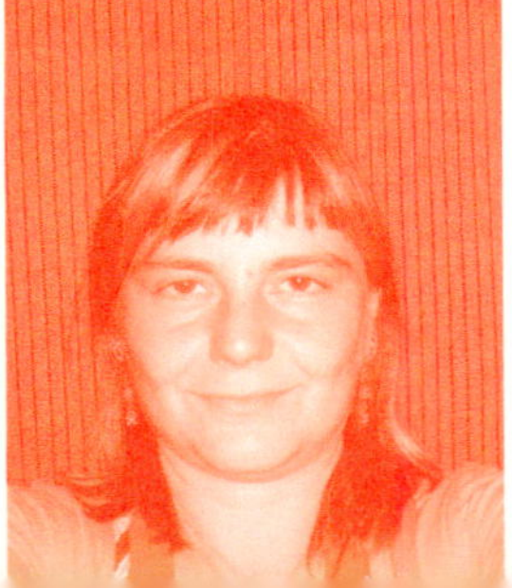

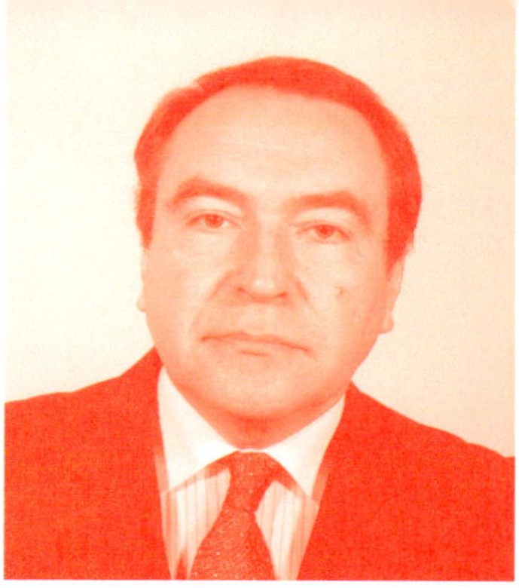
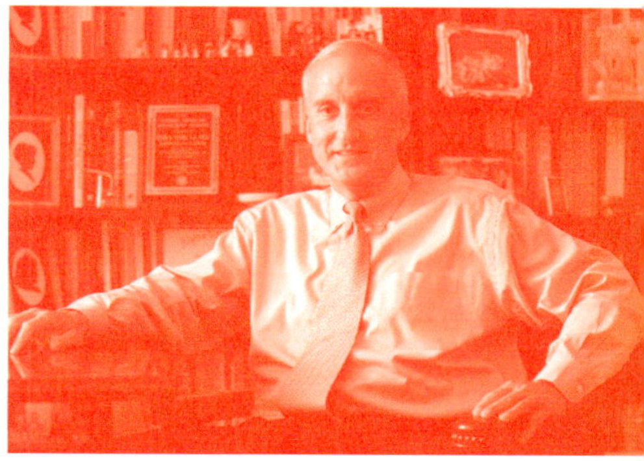
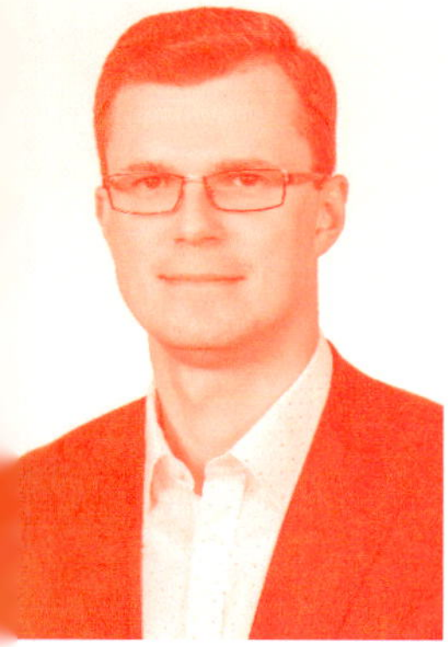
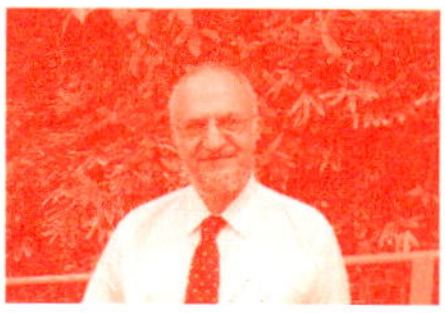
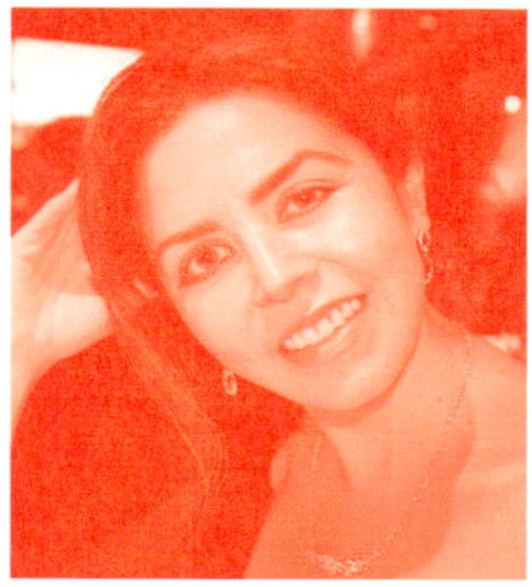

Supporting open minds since 2005

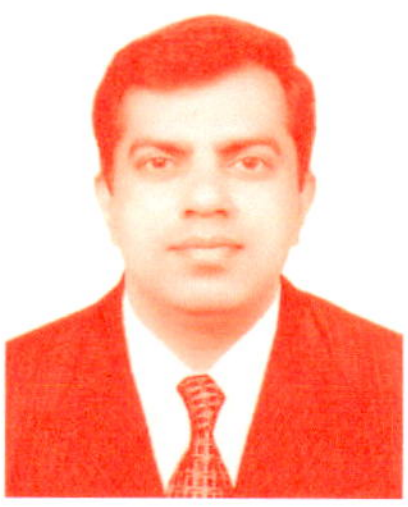
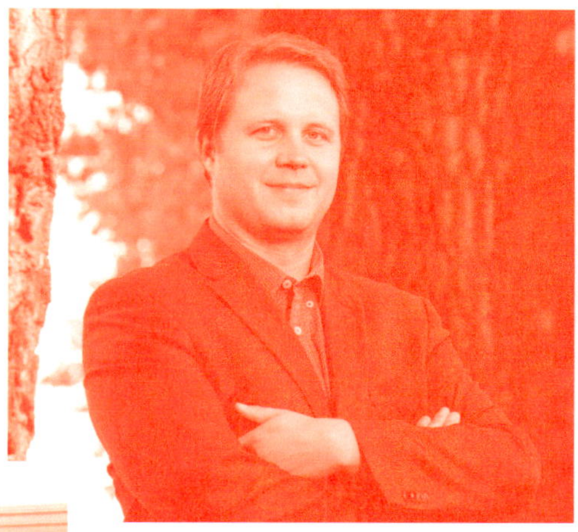
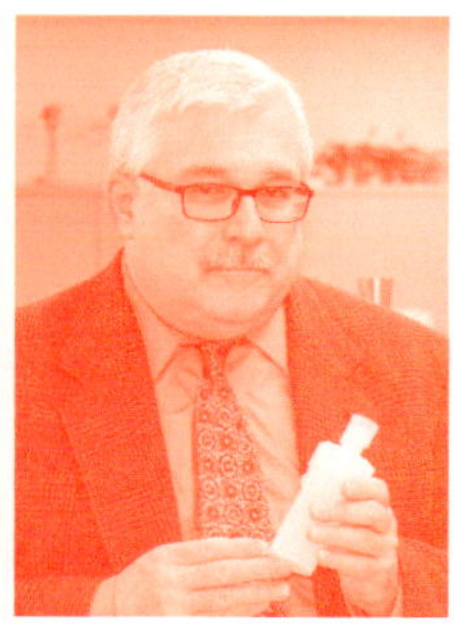
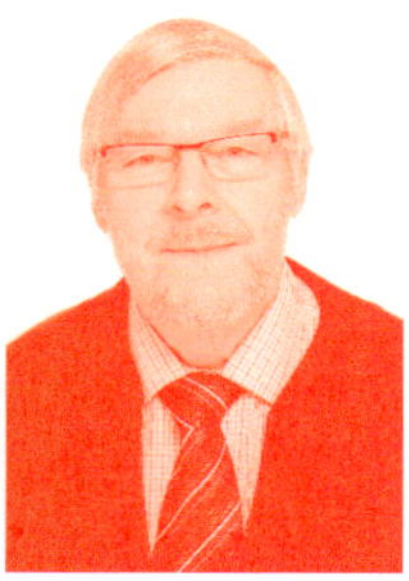
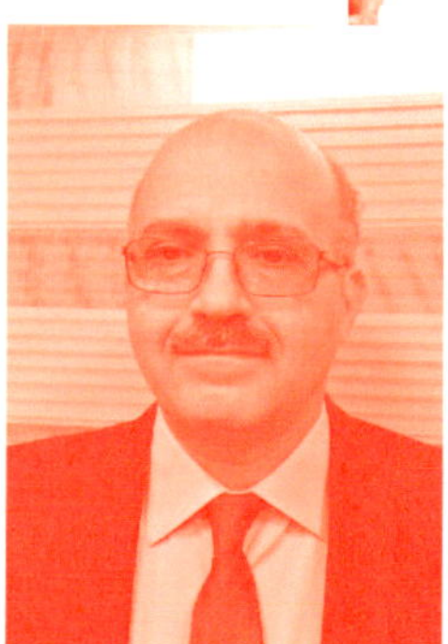
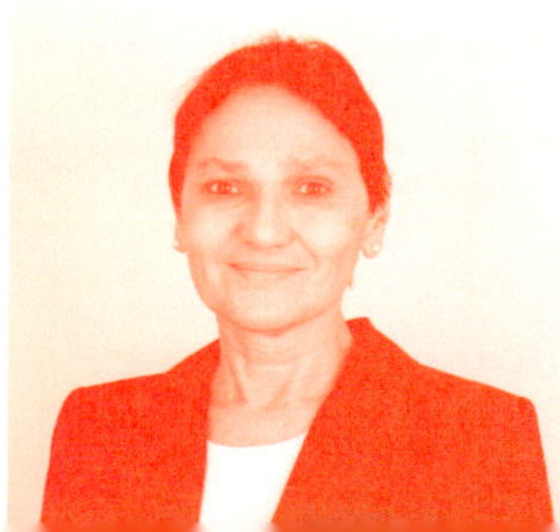
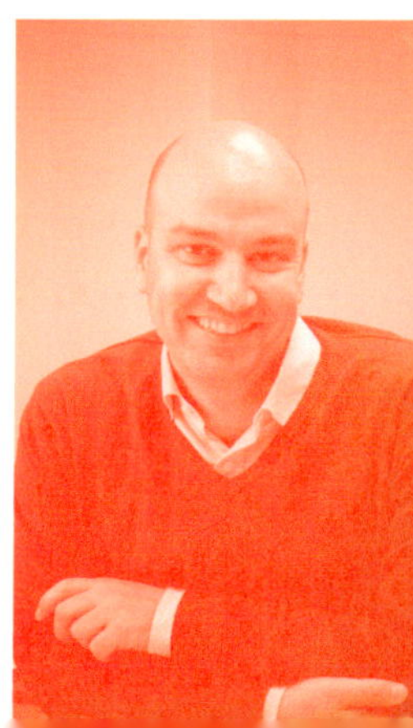

Hypothyroidism - New Aspects of an Old Disease
http://dx.doi.org/10.5772/intechopen.95721
Edited by Ifigenia Kostoglou-Athanassiou

Contributors
Hakan Baş, Fernando Candanedo-Gonzalez, Dafne Noemi Pacheco-Garcilazo, Javier Rios-Valencia, Armando Gamboa-Dominguez, Wilfredo Valenzuela-Gonzalez, Shabnam Heydarzadeh, Mehdi Hedayati, Ali Asghar Moshtaghie, Maryam Daneshpoor, Wissal Abassi, Nejmeddine Ouerghi, Anissa Bouassida, Neha Sharma, Sanghapriya Mukherjee, Aparajita Kushwaha, Ayodeji Folorunsh Ajayi, Emmanuel Tayo Adebayo, Goodness Olusayo Olatinwo, Segun Emmanuel Bamidele, Olubunmi Simeon Oyekunle, Iyanuoluwa Oluwadunsi Adebayo, Victor Oluwaseyi Amos, Shiv Shankar Singh, Prashanjit Laskar, Anindita Deb, Sangita Sutradhar, Christopher L. Lyon Brown, Earl T. Larson, Arjay Pataueg, Ifigenia Kostoglou-Athanassiou, Lambros Athanassiou, Panagiotis Athanassiou

First published in London, United Kingdom, 2022 by IntechOpen
IntechOpen is the global imprint of INTECHOPEN LIMITED, registered in England and Wales, registration number: 11086078, 5 Princes Gate Court, London, SW7 2QJ, United Kingdom
Printed in Croatia

British Library Cataloguing-in-Publication Data
A catalogue record for this book is available from the British Library

Additional hard and PDF copies can be obtained from orders@intechopen.com

Hypothyroidism - New Aspects of an Old Disease
Edited by Ifigenia Kostoglou-Athanassiou
p. cm.
Print ISBN 978-1-83969-340-3
Online ISBN 978-1-83969-341-0
eBook (PDF) ISBN 978-1-83969-342-7

For EU product safety concerns:
IN TECH d.o.o., Prolaz Marije Krucifikse Kozulić 3, 51000 Rijeka, Croatia, info@intechopen.com or visit our website at intechopen.com.

Meet the editor

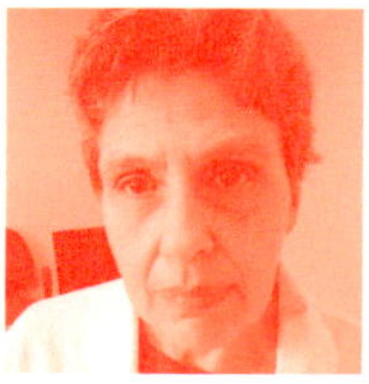

Dr. Ifigenia Kostoglou-Athanassiou was born in Thessaloniki, Greece. She is an endocrinologist who graduated from the Medical School, Aristotle University of Thessaloniki, Greece. She obtained an MD from the University of Athens Medical School, and a Ph.D. from the University of London. Her areas of research include breast cancer, neuroendocrinology, melatonin, thyroid cancer, vitamin D, and autoimmune diseases. She has won several awards for her research. Dr. Kostoglou-Athanassiou has published numerous papers and book chapters. Currently, she works as a consultant endocrinologist and head of the Endocrine Department, Asclepeion Hospital, Voula, Athens, Greece.

Contents

Preface

Hypothyroidism is a common endocrine disorder. It is treated with the synthetic thyroid hormone that mimics the natural hormone produced by the thyroid gland. The disease may be the result of many disorders; however, Hashimoto's thyroiditis is the most common cause. Nowadays, an epidemic of autoimmune diseases may have had an impact on the incidence of Hashimoto's thyroiditis. As such, there is renewed interest in the etiology of Hashimoto's thyroiditis. Moreover, new developments, such as the advent of immune checkpoint inhibitors in the treatment of cancer, have had an impact on the treatment of hypothyroidism in these patients. Therefore, there is renewed interest and new developments in hypothyroidism. This book discusses these advances.

The first section focuses on the etiology and pathogenesis of hypothyroidism. The first chapter in this section discusses different aspects of hypothyroidism and autoimmune thyroiditis with an emphasis on the etiology and pathogenesis of autoimmune Hashimoto's thyroiditis. The second chapter discusses the application of precision medicine tools in the detection, diagnosis, and treatment of thyroid dysfunction. The third chapter reviews different aspects of the morphology of the thyroid gland and the etiology of hypothyroidism. The fourth chapter examines the role of ultrasound in the evaluation of hypothyroidism. The fifth and final chapter in this section describes the role of melatonin in the modulation of thyroid function in an experimental model.

The second section discusses the treatment of hypothyroidism, including severe life-threatening hypothyroidism.

The third section examines the effect of hypothyroidism on various organ systems. The first chapter in this section describes the effect of hypothyroidism on fertility in women. The second chapter discusses the effect of iodine and iodinated amino acids analogous to vertebrate thyroid hormones on sea organisms. The third chapter evaluates glucose metabolism in normal and neoplastic thyroid cells.

This book is the result of the efforts of a group of experts in thyroid physiology and thyroid disease. I gratefully acknowledge the work of the contributing authors. I also wish to thank Kristina Kardum Cvitan and Zrinca Tomicic for their help throughout the publication process.

Last, but not least, I dedicate this book to my mother, Areti, whose example and efforts made it possible for me to become the editor of this book.

Ifigenia Kostoglou-Athanassiou, MSc, MD, Ph.D.
Endocrinologist,
Department of Endocrinology,
Asclepeion Hospital,
Voula, Athens, Greece

Section 1

Hypothyroidism: Etiology and Pathogenesis

Chapter 1

Autoimmune Hashimoto's Thyroiditis and Hypothyroidism: Novel Aspects

Ifigenia Kostoglou-Athanassiou, Lambros Athanassiou and Panagiotis Athanassiou

Abstract

Autoimmune Hashimoto's thyroiditis is an organ specific autoimmune disorder. It affects the thyroid gland and it is characterized by the presence of antibodies to thyroid proteins, namely, thyroid peroxidase, TPOab and thyroglobulin, Tgab and thyroid tissue invasion by lymphocytes. The presence of Hashimoto's thyroiditis may be associated with normal thyroid function or hypothyroidism. In many cases of Hashimoto's thyroiditis with normal thyroid function may progress to subclinical hypothyroidism or overt hypothyroidism. Risk factors for the development of Hashimoto's thyroiditis are genetic and environmental. Genetic factors are HLA-DR4, CD40, CTLA-4 and PTP-N22 and genetic factors related to thyroglobulin gene and TSH receptor gene. Environmental factors include the presence of iodine excess in the environment, infectious agents such as hepatitis C virus and the SARS-CoV-2 virus, smoking, alcohol, selenium deficiency, drugs such as amiodarone, interferon-a, highly active antiretroviral therapy and immune checkpoint inhibitors. Female sex is also a risk factor for Hashimoto's thyroiditis. The disease runs a variable course. Presently there are experimental efforts to pause or reverse the autoimmune process which leads to Hashimoto's thyroiditis and may progress to the destruction of the thyroid gland. Hypothyroidism is treated by the administration of thyroxine usually for life.

Keywords: autoimmune hashimoto's thyroiditis, subclinical hypothyroidism, hypothyroidism, thyroid antibodies, thyroid autoantibodies, thyroxine

1. Introduction

Autoimmune Hashimoto's thyroiditis is a chronic autoimmune thyroid disorder characterized by the presence of goiter in many cases, hypothyroidism in several cases and the presence of antibodies to thyroid antigens in the blood [1–3]. It is a frequent disorder and the most frequent cause of hypothyroidism.

Hashimoto in 1912 described the disease in 4 women who had surgery for goiter and in whom lymphocytic infiltration of the thyroid was observed in the thyroid biopsy [4]. In 1956 Roitt et al. discovered the presence of antithyroid antibodies in these cases [5]. Chronic autoimmune thyroiditis presents mainly with two types of clinical presentation, one presenting with goiter and another presenting with thyroid atrophy and degeneration. Silent and postpartum thyroiditis are two forms of chronic autoimmune thyroiditis.

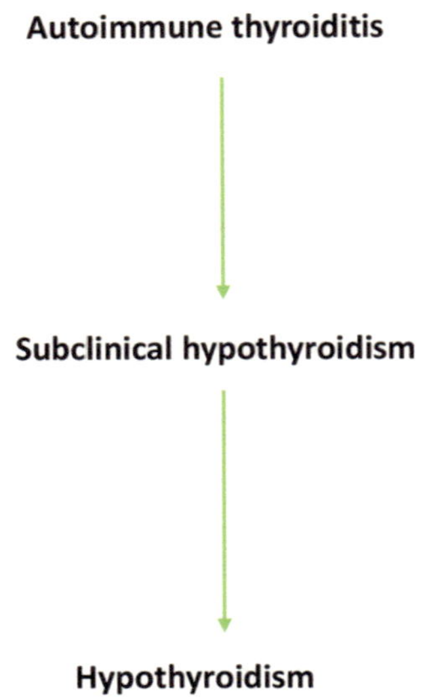

Figure 1.
The progression of autoimmune thyroiditis.

The development of methods for the detection of antithyroid antibodies and measurement of thyroid stimulating hormone (TSH) has led to the diagnosis of cases of chronic autoimmune thyroiditis in patients with normal thyroid function, who in the course of the disease develop subclinical or clinical hypothyroidism (**Figure 1**).

2. Prevalence and incidence

Autoimmune thyroiditis affects 5–7 times more women than men, usually middle aged or older as well as younger patients and children. The prevalence of the disease differs depending on three diagnostic criteria, namely a) the presence of thyroid tissue lymphocytic infiltration b) the detection of antithyroid antibodies, and c) the presence of increased TSH levels.

Foci of thyroiditis 1–10/cm^2 of thyroid tissue in biopsies were observed in 40–45% in females and 20% in males. If the diagnostic limit increases to >40/cm^2 foci of thyroiditis the prevalence is lower, i.e., 5–15% in females and 1–5% in males [6, 7]. The incidence of Hashimoto thyroiditis is 1.3% in children 11–18 years. In adult women the incidence is 3.5 per 1000 per year and in men 0.8 per 1000 per year. Although in a worldwide basis the commonest cause of hypothyroidism remains iodine deficiency, in areas of adequate iodine intake the commonest cause of hypothyroidism is Hashimoto thyroiditis with a worldwide estimated annual incidence of 0.3–1.5 cases per 1000 [8, 9].

The prevalence of positive antithyroid antibodies was investigated in studies performed in Whickham in the UK and in New South Wales in Australia and was 10–13% in female and 5% in male patients [10]. Newer studies however have found a greater incidence of thyroid antibodies which was increasing with age. Vanderpump et al. [9] observed positive thyroglobulin Tgab and thyroid peroxidase TPOab antibodies 10.6 and 14.9% in the age range 18–24 years and 33.3 and 24.2% in the age range of 55–64 years in females, respectively. Mariotti et al. [11] observed 33% positive thyroid antibodies in females aged >70 years. Thyrotropin receptor blocking antibodies, which are antibodies binding and blocking the TSH receptor have been described and may contribute to the development of hypothyroidism [12].

Higher than normal TSH levels in various studies were observed as subclinical hypothyroidism, high TSH and normal T_4, in 3–13.6% in female and 0.7–5.7% in male patients. Clinical hypothyroidism, high TSH and decreased T_4 levels were observed in 0.5–1.9% in females and in <1% of males [10, 13–15]. Canaris et al. [16] in an observational study performed in Colorado, USA, including 25,862 people aged 18–74 years found increased TSH in 9.4% (subclinical 9% and clinical hypothyroidism 0.4%). TSH was 5.1–10 mU/L in 74% of cases and in 26% greater than 10 mU/L. TSH levels were found to increase with age, as they were increased in 4% in the first decade of life and in 21% in the last decade of life in women and in 3% in the first decade of life in male patients and 16% in the last decade in male patients.

The prevalence of chronic autoimmune thyroiditis is better described by the presence of foci of the disease in thyroid tissue and the presence of thyroid antibodies than by TSH levels, which may increase due to other reasons.

3. Pathogenesis

Hashimoto thyroiditis is an autoimmune disorder which may be due to an abnormal immune reaction. T lymphocytes are involved in the pathogenesis of Hashimoto's thyroiditis [17–20] and polycoclonal antibodies are produced targeting thyroid cells. The autoimmune disorder is initiated by the activation of CD4 T helper lymphocytes specific for thyroid antigens [18]. In the literature two hypotheses have been developed for the activation of these cells.

According to the first hypothesis an infection with a virus or a bacterium which has a protein similar to a thyroid protein may induce the activation of T lymphocytes specific for the thyroid, a theory known as theory of molecular mimicry [21, 22]. According to an alternative hypothesis, epithelial thyroid cells present their intracellular proteins to helper T lymphocytes. Following their activation autoreactive CD4 T lymphocytes may stimulate autoreactive B lymphocytes which produce thyroid antibodies. Activated T lymphocytes induce the concentration of cytotoxic CD8 T lymphocytes and B lymphocytes within the thyroid [19]. The direct destruction by T lymphocytes of thyroid cells is believed to be the main mechanism responsible for the development of hypothyroidism. Thyroid antibodies may also play a pathogenetic role.

Increased apoptosis may be involved in the mechanism of thyroid cells destruction in Hashimoto thyroiditis. Cytotoxic T lymphocytes destroy target cells inducing an apoptosis mechanism. Increased apoptosis via Fas-FasL [23, 24] is observed in thyroid cells which are near the infiltrating lymphocytes and this mechanism has been described as a major thyroid cell destruction mechanism in Hashimoto thyroiditis [25].

4. Histology

The form of chronic autoimmune thyroiditis with goiter diffuse lymphocytic and plasmacytic infiltration of the gland takes place with the formation of lymphoid follicles with germinal centers [26, 27]. The changes in the follicular epithelium vary and the most characteristic is the oxyphilic transformation of the cells, known as Hurthle or Eskanazy cells, which may be focal or diffuse with the formation of nodules [28]. The follicular epithelium may be hyperplastic with the formation of papillae or the follicles may be small and atrophic with little colloid and there is fragmentation of their cell walls. Cell nuclei may present with atypia. Histological examination may reveal lymphocytic infiltration and the diagnosis may not be certain, except if high titers of thyroid antibodies are present. In the atrophic form, the thyroid may be small with lymphocytic and plasmacytic infiltration which replace the thyroid parenchyma and fibrosis. It appears that atrophic thyroiditis may be the final stage of that with goiter.

5. Etiology

Various genetic, epigenetic and environmental factors predispose to the development of chronic autoimmune thyroiditis (**Figure 2**).

5.1 Genetic factors

Various genetic factors have been recognized. The genes encoding the major histocompatibility complex HLA have been implicated in the pathogenesis of Hashimoto's thyroiditis [29]. The presence of Tyr26, Gln70, Lys71 and Arg74 in the HLA-DRβ1 molecule may cause structural changes in pocket 4 of the molecule thereby influencing binding of thyroid-derived pathogenic peptides [30] thus predisposing to the development of autoimmune thyroiditis. The presence of Tyr30 in pocket 6 of the HLA-DR molecule may also cause structural changes and predispose to the development of autoimmune thyroiditis [31]. Cytotoxic T lymphocyte associated antigen-4 (CTLA-4) [32] and protein tyrosine phosphatase-22 (PTPN22) [33] are major negative regulators of T cell mediated immune functions. Polymorphisms of the CTLA-4 and PTPN22 genes have been linked with Hashimoto's thyroiditis [32, 33]. However, the mechanisms through which susceptibility to thyroid autoimmunity is induced are yet unknown. The presence of A^{-1623} A/G single-nucleotide polymorphism at the thyroglobulin (Tg) promoter may influence binding of nuclear transcription factors such interferon regulatory factor-1 protein [34]. Increased production of interferon-γ in a viral infection may increase expression of thyroglobulin and lead to activation of T cell response thus leading to the development of thyroid autoimmunity [35]. A polymorphism in the CD40 gene has significant effects on CD40 on antigen-presenting cells, including B lymphocytes, influencing B cell proliferation, antibody secretion and generation of memory cells thus leading to thyroid autoimmunity [36].

5.2 Environmental factors

Infections and iodine are environmental factors which may predispose to the development of Hashimoto's thyroiditis (**Figure 3**). Infectious agents, such hepatitis C virus, may induce autoimmunity by molecular mimicry, tissue infection

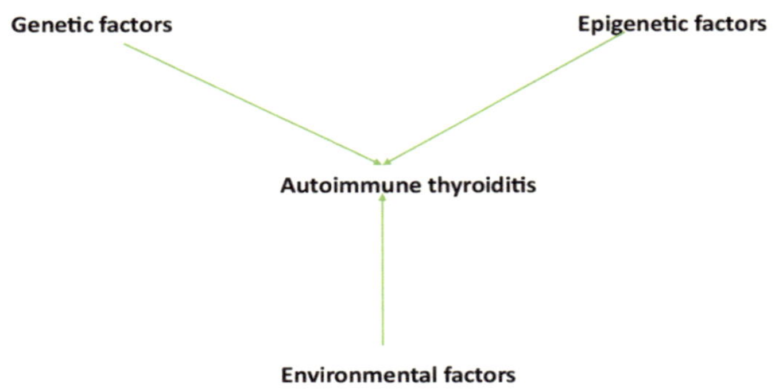

Figure 2.
Factors contributing to the development of autoimmune Hashimoto's thyroiditis.

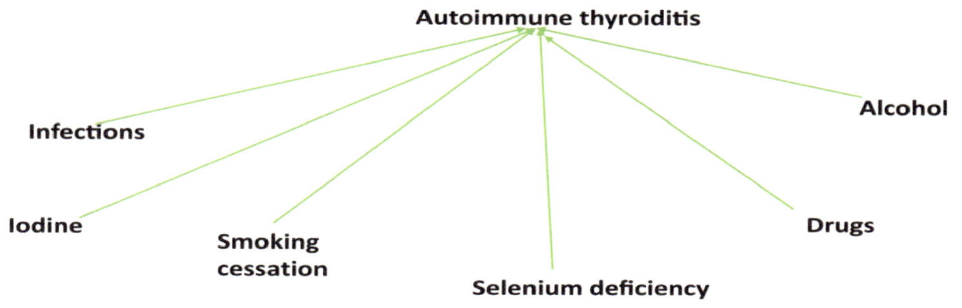

Figure 3.
Environmental risk factors for the development of autoimmune Hashimoto's thyroiditis.

or destruction [37]. An increased prevalence of antithyroid antibodies has been observed in residents in areas with iodine excess [38]. Salt iodination may induce the development of thyroid autoimmunity [39]. The presence of autoimmune thyroiditis has been associated with both iodine deficiency and iodine excess suggesting a U-shaped relationship between iodine status and thyroid autoimmunity risk in adults [40].

5.3 SARS-CoV-2 viral infection

SARS-CoV-2 is a coronavirus which has been related to the development of autoimmunity. Autoimmune thyroid disease, in the form of subacute thyroiditis, autoimmune thyroiditis and Graves' disease have been described in patients with the Covid-19 disease [41, 42]. The development of hypothyroidism following SARS-CoV-2 infection has also been observed.

5.4 Selenium

Selenium deficiency may be related to the development of thyroid autoimmunity [43]. Smoking seems to protect from the development of autoimmune Hashimoto's thyroiditis and hypothyroidism [44]. Smoking cessation leads to loss of protection from autoimmune Hashimoto's thyroiditis. Medium alcohol consumption seems to protect from the development of autoimmune Hashimoto's thyroiditis.

5.5 Estrogens

Autoimmune Hashimoto's thyroiditis has a higher prevalence in female patients [1]. There is a sex dimorphism in the immune response [45]. Female patients have a stronger immune response. The cost is an increased susceptibility to autoimmune diseases [46]. Estrogens modulate the immune response and induce autoimmune diseases [47]. Estrogen withdrawal in menopause also modulates the immune response [48].

5.6 Drugs

Amiodarone has a high iodine content and affects thyroid function. It may induce autoimmune thyroiditis, hypothyroidism or hyperthyroidism [49, 50].

Highly active antiretroviral therapy (HAART) for the treatment of HIV patients is related to a higher incidence of subclinical hypothyroidism [51].

Interferon-α is used for the treatment of hepatitis C and is associated with the development of autoimmune thyroiditis, hypothyroidism and destructive thyroiditis [52].

Immune check point inhibitors are a major step forward in the treatment of cancer. However, their administration is related to the development of autoimmune thyroiditis and autoimmune hypophysitis [53, 54]. In the presence of autoimmune thyroiditis, the requirement for thyroxine treatment increases depicting further immune tissue destruction of the thyroid.

The prevalence of Hashimoto's thyroiditis is increased in relatives of patients with autoimmune thyroiditis, this phenomenon is mostly apparent in first degree relatives. Brix et al. [55] investigated the genetic effect on the etiology of autoimmune thyroid disease in female Danish twins (2945 pairs, 5890 patients) and found that genetic factors affect the incidence of autoimmune thyroid disease.

6. Clinical presentation

The most frequent clinical findings in chronic autoimmune thyroiditis are goiter and hypothyroidism or both.

As far as goiter is concerned, the thyroid is homogenously enlarged, has a semi-hard consistency and its surface is uneven. In some cases, the enlargement is uneven and it may appear as a nodule or multinodular goiter. Rarely, especially in elderly patients, it may present with fibrosis which leads to the diffuse enlargement of the thyroid with hard consistency and the differential diagnosis with malignancy should be performed. Goiter appears gradually and the gland may be enlarged. The thyroid gland is usually minimally enlarged. Generally, there are no symptoms from goiter, except for a feeling of pressure and in very rare cases pain or tenderness on palpation. Very rarely symptoms of pressure of the trachea, the esophagus or the laryngeal nerves may be observed in the case of abrupt enlargement of the thyroid, especially in the case of fibrosis, which need differential diagnosis from thyroid lymphoma or carcinoma. Lymphoma is observed in 0.1% of patients with chronic autoimmune thyroiditis and it is 80 times more frequent than expected [56].

As far as hypothyroidism is concerned, patients with positive antithyroid antibodies are euthyroid in 50-75%, 25-50% have subclinical hypothyroidism and 5–10% have clinical hypothyroidism. Patients with positive antithyroid antibodies and normal or increased TSH, T_4 normal may present with hypothyroidism in the course of the disease. In the Whickham study 20 years later in a group of female patients with normal initial TSH clinical hypothyroidism was observed in 27% and those with increased initial TSH in 55% [9]. This is a finding which indicates that patients with positive thyroid antibodies and normal TSH should be followed up for the development of subclinical or clinical hypothyroidism. In clinical hypothyroidism signs and symptoms of hypothyroidism are observed and the diagnosis is easy. In subclinical hypothyroidism, however, there are no symptoms, although it has been reported that in comparison with euthyroid people there may be symptoms, such as cold intolerance, dry skin, fatigue, depression, disorders of cognition and atypical response to psychiatric intervention [57–59]. Additionally, Canaris et al. [16] comparing the symptoms of hypothyroidism to those of subclinical hypothyroidism, found that the symptoms of patients with subclinical hypothyroidism were intermediate as compared to those of clinical hypothyroidism and those of euthyroid individuals. However, symptoms of subclinical hypothyroidism may be vague and may not be sufficient for the diagnosis of subclinical hypothyroidism, which can be made only by TSH measurement.

7. Diagnosis

For the diagnosis of chronic autoimmune thyroiditis history, clinical presentation and laboratory findings are used.

7.1 History and clinical presentation

The presence of other members of the family with chronic autoimmune thyroiditis will be sought, as the disease may present in families. If there is goiter, the time of presentation will be sought, the size and its change in the course of time, as in thyroiditis the thyroid is gradually enlarged in the course of time. The presence of pressure symptoms will be sought in the trachea and the esophagus. The presence of symptoms of hypothyroidism will also be sought.

Palpation of the thyroid gland will be performed to identify the consistency of the gland, which may be semi-hard and its surface uneven. The findings of hypothyroidism will also be investigated. It should be noted that a rare clinical finding is encephalopathy, Hashimoto' encephalopathy, which regresses either without treatment or by the administration of corticosteroids [60, 61].

7.2 Laboratory findings

Laboratory examination includes biochemical examinations, ultrasonography, thyroid scanning and fine needle aspiration biopsy.

Biochemical examinations: The main characteristic of chronic autoimmune thyroiditis is the presence of positive thyroid antibodies. The titer of TPOab is increased in 95% approximately and those of Tgab in 60% of the cases. Titers of thyroid antibodies are higher in the fibrotic disease than in that with goiter. In micronodular goiter the prevalence of Hashimoto's thyroiditis is increased. Yeh et al. [62] in the presence of micronodules 1–6.5 mm identified positive thyroid antibodies in 94.7% of the cases. Increased thyroid antibodies are observed in other thyroid diseases, as well, but their prevalence is low. In chronic autoimmune thyroiditis usually both TPOab and Tgab are usually present, however, only one type may be present. Takamatsu et al. [63] in their study of 437 patients they observed both types of antibodies present in 316 patients, one type in 85 and none in the rest 36 patients.

In chronic autoimmune thyroiditis antibodies to the TSH receptor are observed. Ducornet et al. [64] in a large review of the literature found TSH-receptor binding-inhibitory immunoglobulins in 9% of patients with thyroiditis and goiter and in 21% in patients with fibrotic atrophic thyroiditis. In the same review they found thyrotropin receptor blocking antibodies in 12% of patients with thyroiditis and goiter and in 33% of patients with atrophic thyroiditis. In patients with hypothyroidism Takasu et al. [65] found thyrotropin receptor blocking antibodies in 10% of patients with thyroiditis and goiter and in 25% of those with atrophic thyroiditis. In newborns with hypothyroidism TSH-receptor binding-inhibitory immunoglobulins were observed in 0.8–38% and in the mothers of those newborns TSH-receptor-binding-inhibitory-immunoglobulins in 5% and thyrotropin receptor blocking antibodies in 4%. These antibodies differ in their action on the TSH receptor. TSH receptor binding inhibitory immunoglobulins bind the receptor, without a stimulating action and they block binding TSH to its receptor. Thyrotropin receptor blocking antibodies block the function of TSH receptor. The presence of these antibodies is important as with thyroxine administration they may disappear and hypothyroidism may regress.

Ultrasonography: The ultrasonogram may be diagnostic of chronic autoimmune thyroiditis, as it gives information on the function of the gland. It reveals increased size of the gland with diffuse hypoechoic areas in 18–77% of cases. Foci of mixed or increased echogenicity may be found in the gland parenchyma, which may be a sign of fibrosis [66, 67]. In some patients many small hypoechoic nodules may be found within the parenchyma of the gland. These nodules present lymphoid tissue or remnants of thyroid follicles and may need to be differentially diagnosed from nodular goiter.

Scanning: Scanning with radioiosotopes does not contribute to the diagnosis of chronic autoimmune thyroiditis and it is not used in everyday practice. If applied it shows nonhomogenous distribution of the radioisotope, a picture like that of multinodular goiter [68]. Radioisotope uptake may be normal or increased in thyroiditis with goiter, even if hypothyroidism is present, and is decreased in subacute thyroiditis or silent thyroiditis.

Fine needle aspiration biopsy: Fine needle aspiration biopsy is not necessary for the diagnosis of chronic autoimmune thyroiditis. It should be performed for the diagnosis of malignancy if goiter increases in size or there are nodules which may be malignant.

Nodules suspicious for malignancy are nodules in the case of a multiglandular familial syndrome, radiation in the head or neck and chest, rapid growth of the nodule, symptoms of local infiltration such as voice hoarseness, dysphagia or dyspnea and if the nodule is hard, irregular, attached to the neighboring tissues or there are enlarged lymph nodes. The possibility of malignancy in a nodule is increased in young and older ages, especially in male patients. Nys et al. [69] in 165 cases of Hashimoto thyroiditis with nodules or pseudonodules found 4% differentiated thyroid cancer and 1% non-Hodgkin's lymphoma. Kumarasinghe and De Silva [70] in 100 patients with autoimmune thyroiditis who had fine needle aspiration biopsy found one case of a papillary and one case of Hurthle cell carcinoma (2%). According to these authors there may be some traps in the diagnosis of the cytologic examination, as in 100 aspiration biopsies the diagnosis was certain in 78 and in the rest 22 it was only suggestive of autoimmune thyroiditis. In the case of the two cancers the typical findings of malignancy were not observed. As potential traps cell atypia, the presence of inflammatory cells either in abundancy or paucity, and the absence of cell abundancy may be observed in autoimmune thyroiditis. The presence of epithelial as opposed to inflammatory cells, the presence of many cell nuclei, intense atypia may suggest malignancy even if the other findings of autoimmune thyroiditis are present. The presence of nuclear atypia as observed in oxyphil cells, in the presence of findings of autoimmune thyroiditis should not suggest the presence of a follicular neoplasm and should not lead to an unnecessary operation.

The diagnosis of chronic autoimmune thyroiditis should be sought for when other autoimmune diseases or other diseases are present, which make its diagnosis possible or probable. Chronic autoimmune thyroiditis has been observed in 70% of patients with multiple endocrine neoplasia type 2C, 50% of people with POEMS syndrome (polyneuropathy, organomegaly, endocrinopathies, M protein and skin alterations), 50% of Turner's syndrome, 20% of Addison's disease, 20% of Down's syndrome and in other diseases such as gastritis, alopecia areata and type 1 diabetes mellitus.

8. Silent and postpartum thyroiditis

Silent and postpartum thyroiditis are thought to be manifestations of chronic autoimmune thyroiditis.

8.1 Silent thyroiditis

Silent thyroiditis is a frequent cause of hyperthyroidism. It is called silent as it does not manifest with pain. It affects equally male and female patients. Hyperthyroidism is mild and there is no history of upper respiratory infection. Hyperthyroidism is due to thyroid hormone release in the blood due to cell lysis and regresses in 6–12 weeks or becomes transient hypothyroidism in 50% of cases which regresses in 2–12 weeks, while in approximately 5% hypothyroidism is permanent. The size of the thyroid is normal or slightly increased and there are no extrathyroidal manifestations of Graves' disease.

Thyroid hormone levels vary depending on the stage of the disease. The most characteristic finding of silent thyroiditis is decreased ^{131}I uptake. TPOab are detected in 60% of cases and Tgab in 25% of cases.

Treatment with antithyroid drugs is not considered necessary as hyperthyroidism is not severe and subsequently hypothyroidism ensues. Beta-blockers may be administered. It should be noted that new episodes of silent thyroiditis may be observed in the future. In long term follow up disease recurrence has been observed in 65% of cases [71].

8.2 Postpartum thyroiditis

Postpartum thyroiditis is frequent. It appears within the first year postpartum and affects 5–10% of female patients. The diagnosis of the disease may not be made as physicians are not aware of the disease and many of the symptoms are thought to be due to depression or other manifestations of the postpartum period. The diagnosis is made by the fact that there is no history of thyroid disorder prior to the pregnancy, there are positive TPoab or Tgab, there are no positive TSH receptor antibodies and there is no toxic adenoma.

In its classical presentation it presents with transient hyperthyroidism usually 6 weeks to 6 months postpartum. Hypothyroidism follows which recedes within the first year postpartum. Its classical presentation refers to 26% of the cases and may present only with hyperthyroidism (38%) or hypothyroidism [72, 73]. Hyperthyroidism is light and of short duration. Treatment is not necessary. If symptoms are present beta-blockers are administered. In the case of hypothyroidism thyroxine treatment is necessary for a period of 6 months. It should be noted that in 25% of cases hypothyroidism is permanent in 4 or more years of follow up [74, 75].

Postpartum thyroiditis is an autoimmune disease. Pregnancy is a period of immunosuppression which is followed by a period of rebound immune activation postpartum. Thus, the titer of thyroid antibodies decreases during pregnancy and may increase in the postpartum period. The highest titer of thyroid antibodies is observed 5–7 months postpartum. Kent et al. [76] studied the prevalence of thyroiditis in 748 female patients 4.5–5.5 months postpartum. They found thyroiditis in 11.5% of the patients and positive TPOab in 63.9% as opposed to 4.9% in female patients without thyroiditis. If thyroid antibodies are present during pregnancy, thyroiditis will be observed in 33–85% of patients [77, 78]. The presence of TPOab affects pregnancy outcome [79].

The most frequent cause of hypothyroidism, which in many cases is subclinical, in pregnancy is thyroid antibodies. Haddow et al. [80] studied 25,216 pregnant patients and found hypothyroidism in 0.25% with positive TPOab in 77%. The children of these patients were studied at the age 7–9 years and none had hypothyroidism, however they presented with neuropsychiatric disorders. The prevalence of hypothyroidism in pregnant patients seems to be even greater. In studies performed in Japan, Belgium and USA in pregnant patients hypothyroidism was observed in 0.3, 2.2, and 2.5% respectively [81–83]. TSH and thyroid antibody measurement should be performed in pregnant patients. TSH measurement should be performed in the first stages of pregnancy as the fetal thyroid is activated within the 12th week of the pregnancy.

9. Treatment

Thyroid antibody titers are not an index of thyroid function and they are not an indication for thyroxine administration, except if there is subclinical or clinical hypothyroidism.

Subclinical hypothyroidism is frequent and in 50% of the cases it is due to autoimmune Hashimoto's thyroiditis. It may also be due to drugs, or other etiology or disorders which increase TSH levels without subclinical hypothyroidism. Initially, it should be confirmed that subclinical hypothyroidism is due to autoimmune thyroiditis. In many cases with increased TSH and positive thyroid antibodies thyroxine should be administered, even if there are no symptoms, due to the risk of progression to clinical hypothyroidism. In the Whickham study [9] 55% of female patients in a follow up period of 20 years progressed to clinical hypothyroidism. The risk is greater in female than male patients and it increases significantly after the age of 45. The frequency of progression to clinical hypothyroidism increases with higher TSH levels and with a higher titer of thyroid antibodies. Several medical colleges and physician bodies agree that subclinical hypothyroidism should be treated if thyroid antibodies are present [84, 85].

Subclinical hypothyroidism which is due to chronic autoimmune thyroiditis should be treated, as there is a risk of progression to clinical hypothyroidism and cholesterol levels are increased. Bindels et al. [15] studied 1191 subjects, aged 40–60 years, and they found subclinical hypothyroidism 1.9% in male and 7.6% in female patients, while 3 male and 3 female patients 0.5% had clinical hypothyroidism. At cholesterol levels less than 193 mg/dl the prevalence of the disease in males was 1.5% and in females 4%, at cholesterol levels 193–309 it was 2 and 8.5% and at cholesterol levels above 309 it was 1.6 and 10.3%, respectively. For an increment of TSH of 1 mU/l cholesterol levels increased in females 3.47 and in males 6.18 mg. Michalopoulou et al. [86] in patients with hypercholesterolemia and TSH in the upper normal range found that thyroxine administration decreased cholesterol levels. The measurement of thyroid hormone levels is important in patients with hypercholesterolemia and in all female patients over the age of 50 years as subclinical hypothyroidism is present in approximately 10%. Cholesterol may increase the risk of coronary artery disease and thyroxine treatment may decrease cholesterol levels and this risk. Despite that, Hak et al. [87] found that in female patients subclinical hypothyroidism is a risk factor for atherosclerosis and cardiac infarction, independently of the levels of cholesterol, HDL cholesterol and smoking. Thyroxine administration in subclinical hypothyroidism should be performed with caution as it may cause tachycardia, atrial fibrillation, and osteoporosis. Thus, thyroxine should be administered with caution especially in elderly patients.

Thyroxine can be administered in its full dose in young patients without cardiac disease. However, in patients with known cardiac disease or in patients aged over 70 years the initial thyroxine dose should be 25 μg daily and should be increased by 25 μg every 4–6 weeks. TSH measurement should be performed every 4 weeks until TSH is within normal range. During follow up thyroid hormones should be measured once a year. Thyroxine dose is approximately 1.6 μg/kg daily and it is age related. Elderly patients need 50% of the adult dose, while children need a higher dose (3.8 μg/kg). In clinical hypothyroidism thyroxine treatment should be initiated with small doses 12.5–25 μg daily and should be increased slowly at monthly intervals. In patients with severe long-standing hypothyroidism or elderly patients caution should be exercised in the initiation of treatment and when the dose is increased. Thyroxine may be administered in liquid or soft gel form. The simultaneous administration of thyroxine and liothyronine for the treatment of hypothyroidism has also been used [88], but it has not been shown to be superior to thyroxine administration. At present, experimental efforts take place to block T cell activation by thyroglobulin by the use of small molecules, such as cepharanathine, in experimentally induced autoimmune thyroiditis and thus stop the progression of the disease [89]. The administration of selenium and vitamin D may interfere with the progression of autoimmune thyroiditis.

Hypothyroidism in chronic autoimmune thyroiditis is not always permanent and there is a percentage of patients who recover and thyroxine may be withdrawn. The recovery of thyroid function is related to decreased titers of thyrotropin receptor blocking antibodies and not to TPOab and Tgab, as these titers do not respond to thyroxine administration. Recovery of thyroid function following thyroxine administration is 0.2–24% with a mean value of 10% [9, 90–93]. In chronic autoimmune thyroiditis thyotropin receptor blocking antibodies are present in approximately 20% [65, 90, 92]. The regression of these antibodies with thyroxine administration does not always lead to the recovery of hypothyroidism. Thyrotropin receptor blocking antibodies decrease in 30–75% of positive patients and recovery of hypothyroidism is observed only in some of these patients [65, 92]. A practical way to test if normal thyroid function is restored is to decrease the dose of thyroxine after a year of treatment and if TSH levels remain normal to withdraw thyroxine. Following thyroxine withdrawal TSH should be measured 4–6 weeks later. If TSH levels are normal thyroxine administration should be discontinued and the patient should be followed up. Goiter size decreases with thyroxine administration in patients with chronic autoimmune thyroiditis. It is decreased by 1/3 in 50–90% of patients after a period of 6 months on thyroxine treatment.

10. Conclusion

In conclusion, chronic autoimmune thyroiditis or Hashimoto's thyroiditis is a frequent endocrine disorder which affects more female than male patients. It has been observed after SARS-CoV-2 infection. It frequently causes hypothyroidism. The effects of hypothyroidism decrease quality of life. Its diagnosis is important and should be performed promptly. Thyroid hormones should be measured in female patients after the age of 50 years, in pregnant patients and in the postpartum period and in male patients with hypercholesterolemia. Treatment of hypothyroidism is performed with thyroxine. Thyroxine in the form of liquid or soft gel preparation may also be used. There are efforts to inhibit the autoimmune process in Hashimoto thyroiditis by small molecules, however these efforts have not yet been applied in clinical practice. Treatment with thyroxine is long term and usually for life.

Author details

Ifigenia Kostoglou-Athanassiou[1]*, Lambros Athanassiou[2] and Panagiotis Athanassiou[3]

1 Department of Endocrinology, Asclepeion Hospital, Voula, Athens, Greece

2 Department of Rheumatology, Asclepeion Hospital, Voula, Athens, Greece

3 Department of Rheumatology, St. Paul's Hospital, Thessaloniki, Greece

*Address all correspondence to: ikostoglouathanassiou@yahoo.gr

References

[1] Hiromatsu Y, Satoh H, Amino N. Hashimoto's thyroiditis: History and future outlook. Hormones (Athens, Greece). 2013;**12**(1):12-18. DOI: 10.1007/bf03401282

[2] Ralli M, Angeletti D, Fiore M, et al. Hashimoto's thyroiditis: An update on pathogenic mechanisms, diagnostic protocols, therapeutic strategies, and potential malignant transformation. Autoimmunity Reviews. 2020;**19**(10): 102649. DOI: 10.1016/j.autrev.2020. 102649

[3] Caturegli P, De Remigis A, Rose NR. Hashimoto thyroiditis: Clinical and diagnostic criteria. Autoimmunity Reviews. 2014;**13**(4-5):391-397. DOI: 10.1016/j.autrev.2014.01.007

[4] Hashimoto H. Zur kenntnis der lymphomatosen Veranderung der Sshilddruse (Struma lymphomatosa). Arch Klin Chir. 1912;**97**:219-248

[5] Roitt IM, Campbell PN, Doniach D. The nature of the thyroid auto-antibodies present in patients with Hashimoto's thyroiditis (lymphadenoid goitre). The Biochemical Journal. 1958;**69**(2):248-256. DOI: 10.1042/bj0690248

[6] Williams ED, Doniach I. The post-mortem incidence of focal thyroiditis. The Journal of Pathology and Bacteriology. 1962;**83**:255-264. DOI: 10.1002/path.1700830127

[7] Okayasu I, Hara Y, Nakamura K, Rose NR. Racial and age-related differences in incidence and severity of focal autoimmune thyroiditis. American Journal of Clinical Pathology. 1994;**101**(6):698-702. DOI: 10.1093/ ajcp/101.6.698

[8] Vanderpump MP. The epidemiology of thyroid disease. British Medical Bulletin. 2011;**99**:39-51. DOI: 10.1093/ bmb/ldr030

[9] Vanderpump MP, Tunbridge WM, French JM, et al. The incidence of thyroid disorders in the community: A twenty-year follow-up of the Whickham Survey. Clinical Endocrinology. 1995;**43**(1):55-68. DOI: 10.1111/j.1365-2265.1995.tb01894.x

[10] Tunbridge WM, Evered DC, Hall R, et al. The spectrum of thyroid disease in a community: The Whickham survey. Clinical Endocrinology. 1977;**7**(6):481-493. DOI: 10.1111/j.1365-2265.1977. tb01340.x

[11] Mariotti S, Sansoni P, Barbesino G, et al. Thyroid and other organ-specific autoantibodies in healthy centenarians. Lancet. 1992;**339**(8808):1506-1508. DOI: 10.1016/0140-6736(92)91265-a

[12] Diana T, Krause J, Olivo PD, et al. Prevalence and clinical relevance of thyroid stimulating hormone receptor-blocking antibodies in autoimmune thyroid disease. Clinical and Experimental Immunology. 2017;**189**(3):304-309. DOI: 10.1111/ cei.12980

[13] Sawin CT, Castelli WP, Hershman JM, McNamara P, Bacharach P. The aging thyroid. Thyroid deficiency in the Framingham Study. Archives of Internal Medicine. 1985;**145**(8):1386-1388

[14] Konno N, Yuri K, Taguchi H, et al. Screening for thyroid diseases in an iodine sufficient area with sensitive thyrotrophin assays, and serum thyroid autoantibody and urinary iodide determinations. Clinical Endocrinology. 1993;**38**(3):273-281. DOI: 10.1111/j.1365-2265.1993.tb01006.x

[15] Bindels AJ, Westendorp RG, Frölich M, Seidell JC, Blokstra A, Smelt AH. The prevalence of subclinical hypothyroidism at different total plasma cholesterol levels in middle aged men

and women: A need for case-finding? Clinical Endocrinology. 1999;**50**(2): 217-220. DOI: 10.1046/j.1365-2265. 1999.00638.x

[16] Canaris GJ, Manowitz NR, Mayor G, Ridgway EC. The Colorado thyroid disease prevalence study. Archives of Internal Medicine. 2000;**160**(4):526-534. DOI: 10.1001/archinte.160.4.526

[17] Pyzik A, Grywalska E, Matyjaszek-Matuszek B, Roliński J. Immune disorders in Hashimoto's thyroiditis: What do we know so far? Journal of Immunology Research. 2015;**2015**:979167. DOI: 10.1155/ 2015/979167

[18] Cui X, Liu Y, Wang S, et al. Circulating exosomes activate dendritic cells and induce unbalanced CD4+ T cell differentiation in hashimoto thyroiditis. The Journal of Clinical Endocrinology and Metabolism. 2019;**104**(10):4607-4618. DOI: 10.1210/jc.2019-00273

[19] del Prete GF, Maggi E, Mariotti S, et al. Cytolytic T lymphocytes with natural killer activity in thyroid infiltrate of patients with Hashimoto's thyroiditis: Analysis at clonal level. The Journal of Clinical Endocrinology and Metabolism. 1986;**62**(1):52-57. DOI: 10.1210/jcem-62-1-52

[20] Del Prete GF, Vercelli D, Tiri A, et al. In vivo activated cytotoxic T cells in the thyroid infiltrate of patients with Hashimoto's thyroiditis. Clinical and Experimental Immunology. 1986;**65**(1): 140-147

[21] Benvenga S, Guarneri F. Molecular mimicry and autoimmune thyroid disease. Reviews in Endocrine & Metabolic Disorders. 2016;**17**(4):485-498. DOI: 10.1007/s11154-016-9363-2

[22] Cuan-Baltazar Y, Soto-Vega E. Microorganisms associated to thyroid autoimmunity. Autoimmunity Reviews. 2020;**19**(9):102614. DOI: 10.1016/j. autrev.2020.102614

[23] Abe Y. Apoptosis in the pathogenesis of autoimmune thyroid disease. Nihon Rinsho. 1999;**57**(8):1717-1722

[24] Stassi G, Todaro M, Bucchieri F, et al. Fas/Fas ligand-driven T cell apoptosis as a consequence of ineffective thyroid immunoprivilege in Hashimoto's thyroiditis. Journal of Immunology. 1999;**162**(1):263-267

[25] Phelps E, Wu P, Bretz J, Baker JR Jr. Thyroid cell apoptosis. A new understanding of thyroid autoimmunity. Endocrinology and Metabolism Clinics of North America. 2000;**29**(2):375-388. DOI: 10.1016/ s0889-8529(05)70137-7

[26] Akamizu T, Amino N. Hashimoto's thyroiditis. In: Feingold KR, Anawalt B, Boyce A, et al., editors. Endotext. Oregon, USA: MDText.com, Inc; 2000

[27] Mohr A, Trésallet C, Monot N, et al. Tissue infiltrating LTi-like group 3 innate lymphoid cells and T follicular helper cells in Graves' and Hashimoto's thyroiditis. Frontiers in Immunology. 2020;**11**:601. DOI: 10.3389/ fimmu.2020.00601

[28] Müller-Höcker J. Expression of bcl-2, bax and fas in oxyphil cells of Hashimoto thyroiditis. Virchows Archiv. 2000;**436**(6):602-607. DOI: 10.1007/ s004280000188

[29] Weissel M, Höfer R, Zasmeta H, Mayr WR. HLA-DR and Hashimoto's thyroiditis. Tissue Antigens. 1980;**16**(3): 256-257. DOI: 10.1111/j.1399-0039.1980. tb00302.x

[30] Menconi F, Monti MC, Greenberg DA, et al. Molecular amino acid signatures in the MHC class II peptide-binding pocket predispose to autoimmune thyroiditis in humans and in mice. Proceedings of the National Academy of Sciences of the United States of America. 2008;**105**(37):14034-14039. DOI: 10.1073/pnas.0806584105

[31] Li CW, Osman R, Menconi F, Concepcion ES, Tomer Y. Flexible peptide recognition by HLA-DR triggers specific autoimmune T-cell responses in autoimmune thyroiditis and diabetes. Journal of Autoimmunity. 2017;**76**:1-9. DOI: 10.1016/j.jaut.2016.09.007

[32] Hu Y, Xu K, Jiang L, Zhang L, Shi H, Cui D. Associations between three CTLA-4 polymorphisms and Hashimoto's thyroiditis risk: An updated meta-analysis with trial sequential analysis. Genetic Testing and Molecular Biomarkers. 2018;**22**(4):224-236. DOI: 10.1089/gtmb.2017.0243

[33] Xiaoheng C, Yizhou M, Bei H, et al. General and specific genetic polymorphism of cytokines-related gene in AITD. Mediators of Inflammation. 2017;**2017**:3916395. DOI: 10.1155/2017/3916395

[34] Lahooti H, Edirimanne S, Walsh JP, Delbridge L, Hibbert EJ, Wall JR. Single nucleotide polymorphism 1623 A/G (rs180195) in the promoter of the Thyroglobulin gene is associated with autoimmune thyroid disease but not with thyroid ophthalmopathy. Clinical Ophthalmology. 2017;**11**:1337-1345. DOI: 10.2147/opth.s136070

[35] Stefan M, Jacobson EM, Huber AK, et al. Novel variant of thyroglobulin promoter triggers thyroid autoimmunity through an epigenetic interferon alpha-modulated mechanism. The Journal of Biological Chemistry. 2011;**286**(36):31168-31179. DOI: 10.1074/jbc.M111.247510

[36] Jacobson EM, Tomer Y. The CD40, CTLA-4, thyroglobulin, TSH receptor, and PTPN22 gene quintet and its contribution to thyroid autoimmunity: Back to the future. Journal of Autoimmunity. 2007;**28**(2-3):85-98. DOI: 10.1016/j.jaut.2007.02.006

[37] Hammerstad SS, Blackard JT, Lombardi A, et al. Hepatitis C virus infection of human thyrocytes: Metabolic, hormonal, and immunological implications. The Journal of Clinical Endocrinology and Metabolism. 2020;**105**(4):1157-1168. DOI: 10.1210/clinem/dgz241

[38] Farebrother J, Zimmermann MB, Andersson M. Excess iodine intake: Sources, assessment, and effects on thyroid function. Annals of the New York Academy of Sciences. 2019;**1446**(1):44-65. DOI: 10.1111/nyas.14041

[39] Teti C, Panciroli M, Nazzari E, et al. Iodoprophylaxis and thyroid autoimmunity: An update. Immunologic Research. 2021;**69**(2):129-138. DOI: 10.1007/s12026-021-09192-6

[40] Wang B, He W, Li Q, et al. U-shaped relationship between iodine status and thyroid autoimmunity risk in adults. European Journal of Endocrinology. 2019;**181**(3):255-266. DOI: 10.1530/eje-19-0212

[41] Speer G, Somogyi P. Thyroid complications of SARS and coronavirus disease 2019 (COVID-19). Endocrine Journal. 2021;**68**(2):129-136. DOI: 10.1507/endocrj.EJ20-0443

[42] Brancatella A, Ricci D, Viola N, Sgrò D, Santini F, Latrofa F. Subacute Thyroiditis After Sars-COV-2 Infection. The Journal of Clinical Endocrinology & Metabolism. 2020;**105**(7):dgaa276. DOI: 10.1210/clinem/dgaa276

[43] Ventura M, Melo M, Carrilho F. Selenium and thyroid disease: From pathophysiology to treatment. International Journal of Endocrinology. 2017;**2017**:1297658. DOI: 10.1155/2017/1297658

[44] Sawicka-Gutaj N, Gutaj P, Sowiński J, et al. Influence of cigarette smoking on thyroid gland—An update. Endokrynologia Polska. 2014;**65**(1):54-62. DOI: 10.5603/ep.2014.0008

[45] Taneja V. Sex hormones determine immune response. Frontiers in Immunology. 2018;**9**:1931. DOI: 10.3389/fimmu.2018.01931

[46] Moulton VR. Sex hormones in acquired immunity and autoimmune disease. Frontiers in Immunology. 2018;**9**:2279. DOI: 10.3389/fimmu.2018.02279

[47] Kovats S. Estrogen receptors regulate innate immune cells and signaling pathways. Cellular Immunology. 2015;**294**(2):63-69. DOI: 10.1016/j.cellimm.2015.01.018

[48] Sárvári M, Kalló I, Hrabovszky E, Solymosi N, Liposits Z. Ovariectomy and subsequent treatment with estrogen receptor agonists tune the innate immune system of the hippocampus in middle-aged female rats. PLoS One. 2014;**9**(2):e88540. DOI: 10.1371/journal.pone.0088540

[49] Trohman RG, Sharma PS, McAninch EA, Bianco AC. Amiodarone and thyroid physiology, pathophysiology, diagnosis and management. Trends in Cardiovascular Medicine. 2019;**29**(5):285-295. DOI: 10.1016/j.tcm.2018.09.005

[50] Jabrocka-Hybel A, Bednarczuk T, Bartalena L, et al. Amiodarone and the thyroid. Endokrynologia Polska. 2015;**66**(2):176-186. DOI: 10.5603/ep.2015.0025

[51] Madeddu G, Spanu A, Chessa F, et al. Thyroid function in human immunodeficiency virus patients treated with highly active antiretroviral therapy (HAART): A longitudinal study. Clinical Endocrinology. 2006;**64**(4):375-383. DOI: 10.1111/j.1365-2265.2006.02472.x

[52] Prummel MF, Laurberg P. Interferon-alpha and autoimmune thyroid disease. Thyroid. 2003;**13**(6):547-551. DOI: 10.1089/105072503322238809

[53] Ferrari SM, Fallahi P, Galetta F, Citi E, Benvenga S, Antonelli A. Thyroid disorders induced by checkpoint inhibitors. Reviews in Endocrine & Metabolic Disorders. 2018;**19**(4):325-333. DOI: 10.1007/s11154-018-9463-2

[54] González-Rodríguez E, Rodríguez-Abreu D. Immune checkpoint inhibitors: Review and management of endocrine adverse events. The Oncologist. 2016;**21**(7):804-816. DOI: 10.1634/theoncologist.2015-0509

[55] Brix TH, Hegedüs L. Twins as a tool for evaluating the influence of genetic susceptibility in thyroid autoimmunity. Annales d'endocrinologie. 2011;**72**(2):103-107. DOI: 10.1016/j.ando.2011.03.013

[56] Kato I, Tajima K, Suchi T, et al. Chronic thyroiditis as a risk factor of B-cell lymphoma in the thyroid gland. Japanese Journal of Cancer Research. 1985;**76**(11):1085-1090

[57] Haggerty JJ Jr, Garbutt JC, Evans DL, et al. Subclinical hypothyroidism: A review of neuropsychiatric aspects. International Journal of Psychiatry in Medicine. 1990;**20**(2):193-208. DOI: 10.2190/adly-1uu0-1a8l-hpxy

[58] Haggerty JJ Jr, Stern RA, Mason GA, Marquardt M, Prange AJ Jr. Subclinical hypothyroidism: Recognition, significance, management. Clinical Neuropharmacology. 1992;**15** (Suppl. 1 Pt A):386a. DOI: 10.1097/00002826-199201001-00201

[59] Jackson IM. The thyroid axis and depression. Thyroid. 1998;**8**(10):951-956. DOI: 10.1089/thy.1998.8.951

[60] Mocellin R, Walterfang M, Velakoulis D. Hashimoto's encephalopathy: Epidemiology, pathogenesis and management. CNS Drugs. 2007;**21**(10):799-811. DOI: 10.2165/00023210-200721100-00002

[61] Churilov LP, Sobolevskaia PA, Stroev YI. Thyroid gland and brain: Enigma of Hashimoto's encephalopathy. Best Practice & Research. Clinical Endocrinology & Metabolism. 2019;**33**(6):101364. DOI: 10.1016/j.beem.2019.101364

[62] Yeh HC, Futterweit W, Gilbert P. Micronodulation: Ultrasonographic sign of Hashimoto thyroiditis. Journal of Ultrasound in Medicine. 1996;**15**(12):813-819. DOI: 10.7863/jum.1996.15.12.813

[63] Takamatsu J, Yoshida S, Yokozawa T, et al. Correlation of antithyroglobulin and antithyroid-peroxidase antibody profiles with clinical and ultrasound characteristics of chronic thyroiditis. Thyroid. 1998;**8**(12):1101-1106. DOI: 10.1089/thy.1998.8.1101

[64] Ducornet B, Moisson-Meer A, Duprey J. Hypothyroidism and blocking antibodies. Annales de medecine interne (Paris). 1995;**146**(8):559-574

[65] Takasu N, Yamada T, Takasu M, et al. Disappearance of thyrotropin-blocking antibodies and spontaneous recovery from hypothyroidism in autoimmune thyroiditis. The New England Journal of Medicine. 1992;**326**(8):513-518. DOI: 10.1056/nejm199202203260803

[66] Nordmeyer JP, Shafeh TA, Heckmann C. Thyroid sonography in autoimmune thyroiditis. A prospective study on 123 patients. Acta Endocrinologica. 1990;**122**(3):391-395. DOI: 10.1530/acta.0.1220391

[67] Sostre S, Reyes MM. Sonographic diagnosis and grading of Hashimoto's thyroiditis. Journal of Endocrinological Investigation. 1991;**14**(2):115-121. DOI: 10.1007/bf03350281

[68] Ramtoola S, Maisey MN, Clarke SE, Fogelman I. The thyroid scan in Hashimoto's thyroiditis: The great mimic. Nuclear Medicine Communications. 1988;**9**(9):639-645. DOI: 10.1097/00006231-198809000-00006

[69] Nys P, Merceron RE, Cordray JP, et al. Nodular or pseudo-nodular Hashimoto thyroiditis. Value of cytologic examination. La Presse médicale. 1995;**24**(14):675-678 Thyroïdites de hashimoto à aspect nodulaire ou pseudo-nodulaire. Intérêt de l'examen cytologique

[70] Kumarasinghe MP, De Silva S. Pitfalls in cytological diagnosis of autoimmune thyroiditis. Pathology. 1999;**31**(1):1-7. DOI: 10.1080/003130299105430

[71] Ozawa Y. Painless (silent) thyroiditis. Nihon Rinsho. 1999;**57**(8):1770-1774

[72] Stagnaro-Green A. Postpartum thyroiditis. Best Practice & Research. Clinical Endocrinology & Metabolism. 2004;**18**(2):303-316. DOI: 10.1016/j.beem.2004.03.008

[73] Stagnaro-Green A, Abalovich M, Alexander E, et al. Guidelines of the American Thyroid Association for the diagnosis and management of thyroid disease during pregnancy and postpartum. Thyroid. 2011;**21**(10):1081-1125. DOI: 10.1089/thy.2011.0087

[74] Tachi J, Amino N, Tamaki H, Aozasa M, Iwatani Y, Miyai K. Long term follow-up and HLA association in patients with postpartum hypothyroidism. The Journal of Clinical Endocrinology and Metabolism. 1988;**66**(3):480-484. DOI: 10.1210/jcem-66-3-480

[75] Othman S, Phillips DI, Parkes AB, et al. A long-term follow-up of postpartum thyroiditis. Clinical Endocrinology. 1990;**32**(5):559-564. DOI: 10.1111/j.1365-2265.1990.tb00898.x

[76] Kent GN, Stuckey BG, Allen JR, Lambert T, Gee V. Postpartum thyroid dysfunction: Clinical assessment and relationship to psychiatric affective morbidity. Clinical Endocrinology. 1999;**51**(4):429-438. DOI: 10.1046/j.1365-2265.1999.00807.x

[77] Vargas MT, Briones-Urbina R, Gladman D, Papsin FR, Walfish PG. Antithyroid microsomal autoantibodies and HLA-DR5 are associated with postpartum thyroid dysfunction: Evidence supporting an autoimmune pathogenesis. The Journal of Clinical Endocrinology and Metabolism. 1988;**67**(2):327-333. DOI: 10.1210/jcem-67-2-327

[78] Gerstein HC. How common is postpartum thyroiditis? A methodologic overview of the literature. Archives of Internal Medicine. 1990;**150**(7):1397-1400

[79] Meena A, Nagar P. Pregnancy outcome in euthyroid women with anti-thyroid peroxidase antibodies. Journal of Obstetrics and Gynaecology of India. 2016;**66**(3):160-165. DOI: 10.1007/s13224-014-0657-6

[80] Haddow JE, Palomaki GE, Allan WC, et al. Maternal thyroid deficiency during pregnancy and subsequent neuropsychological development of the child. New England Journal of Medicine. 1999;**341**(8):549-555. DOI: 10.1056/nejm199908193410801

[81] Kamijo K, Saito T, Sato M, et al. Transient subclinical hypothyroidism in early pregnancy. Endocrinologia Japonica. 1990;**37**(3):397-403. DOI: 10.1507/endocrj1954.37.397

[82] Klein RZ, Haddow JE, Faix JD, et al. Prevalence of thyroid deficiency in pregnant women. Clinical Endocrinology. 1991;**35**(1):41-46. DOI: 10.1111/j.1365-2265.1991.tb03494.x

[83] Glinoer D. Maternal thyroid function in pregnancy. Journal of Endocrinological Investigation. 1993;**16**(5):374-378. DOI: 10.1007/bf03348861

[84] Sue LY, Leung AM. Levothyroxine for the treatment of subclinical hypothyroidism and cardiovascular disease. Frontiers in Endocrinology (Lausanne). 2020;**11**:591588. DOI: 10.3389/fendo.2020.591588

[85] Biondi B, Cappola AR, Cooper DS. Subclinical hypothyroidism: A Review. Journal of the American Medical Association. 2019;**322**(2):153-160. DOI: 10.1001/jama.2019.9052

[86] Michalopoulou G, Alevizaki M, Piperingos G, et al. High serum cholesterol levels in persons with 'high-normal' TSH levels: Should one extend the definition of subclinical hypothyroidism? European Journal of Endocrinology. 1998;**138**(2):141-145. DOI: 10.1530/eje.0.1380141

[87] Hak AE, Pols HA, Visser TJ, Drexhage HA, Hofman A, Witteman JC. Subclinical hypothyroidism is an independent risk factor for atherosclerosis and myocardial infarction in elderly women: The Rotterdam Study. Annals of Internal Medicine. 2000;**132**(4):270-278. DOI: 10.7326/0003-4819-132-4-200002150-00004

[88] Jonklaas J, Bianco AC, Cappola AR, et al. Evidence-based use of levothyroxine/liothyronine combinations in treating hypothyroidism: A consensus document. Thyroid. 2021;**31**(2):156-182. DOI: 10.1089/thy.2020.0720

[89] Li CW, Menconi F, Osman R, et al. Identifying a small molecule blocking antigen presentation in autoimmune thyroiditis. The Journal of Biological Chemistry. 2016;**291**(8):4079-4090. DOI: 10.1074/jbc.M115.694687

[90] Rieu M, Richard A, Rosilio M, et al. Effects of thyroid status on thyroid autoimmunity expression in euthyroid and hypothyroid patients with Hashimoto's thyroiditis. Clinical Endocrinology. 1994;**40**(4):529-535. DOI: 10.1111/j.1365-2265.1994.tb02494.x

[91] Battelino T, Krzisnik C, Gottschalk ME, Zeller WP. Testing for thyroid function recovery in children and adolescents with Hashimoto thyroiditis. Annals of Clinical and Laboratory Science. 1994;**24**(6):489-494

[92] Khoo DH, Eng PH, Ho SC, Fok AC. Differences in the levels of TSH-binding inhibitor immunoglobulins in goitrous and agoitrous autoimmune thyroiditis after twelve months of L-thyroxine therapy. Clinical Endocrinology. 1999;**51**(1):73-79. DOI: 10.1046/j.1365-2265.1999.00740.x

[93] Comtois R, Faucher L, Laflèche L. Outcome of hypothyroidism caused by Hashimoto's thyroiditis. Archives of Internal Medicine. 1995;**155**(13):1404-1408

Chapter 2

Application of Data Science Approaches to Investigate Autoimmune Thyroid Disease in Precision Medicine

Ayodeji Folorunsho Ajayi, Emmanuel Tayo Adebayo, Iyanuoluwa Oluwadunsi Adebayo, Olubunmi Simeon Oyekunle, Victor Oluwaseyi Amos, Segun Emmanuel Bamidele and Goodness Olusayo Olatinwo

Abstract

In recent times, the application of artificial intelligence in facilitating, capturing, and restructuring Big data has transformed the accuracy of diagnosis and treatment of diseases, a field known as precision medicine. Big data has been established in various domains of medicine for example, artificial intelligence has found its way into immunology termed as immunoinformatics. There is evidence that precision medicine tools have made an effort to accurately detect, profile, and suggest treatment regimens for thyroid dysfunction using Big data such as imaging and genetic sequences. In addition, the accumulation of data on polymorphisms, autoimmune thyroid disease, and genetic data related to environmental factors has occurred over time resulting in drastic development of clinical autoimmune thyroid disease study. This review emphasized how genetic data plays a vital role in diagnosing and treating diseases related to autoimmune thyroid disease like Graves' disease, subtle subclinical thyroid dysfunctions, Hashimoto's thyroiditis, and hypothyroid autoimmune thyroiditis. Furthermore, connotation between environmental and endocrine risk factors in the etiology of the disease in genetically susceptible individuals were discussed. Thus, endocrinologists' potential hurdles in cancer and thyroid nodules field include unreliable biomarkers, lack of distinct therapeutic alternatives due to genetic difference. Precision medicine data may improve their diagnostic and therapeutic capabilities using artificial intelligence.

Keywords: artificial intelligence, autoimmune disease, Big data, Graves' disease, precision medicine, thyroid disease

1. Introduction

A breakthrough was launched for the field of personalized medicine when the president of the United States of America announced precision medicine in January

2015, presenting it for review and implementation by all healthcare professionals [1]. Since then, molecular characterization of patients which are more precise has been developed in the area which includes an increasing number of 'omics': (proteomics, genomics, transcriptomics, lipidomics, metabolomics and epigenomics), integration of genomic data, the rapid exchange of knowledge among researchers, bioinformatics which involves the retrieval and analysis of data stored in the large databases, and the growing world of Big data and artificial intelligence [1, 2]. These factors are introduced to drive clinicians towards diagnosis, follow-up and therapeutic decisions in precision medicine [2].

Data science applies the use of machine learning algorithms to audio, video, images, text, and numbers to develop artificial intelligence (AI) systems which are used in data processing and preparation of analysis, optimization and construction of integral models, which is further used in the combination of certain algorithm and consequently produce insights that analysts can translate to add value to existing knowledge [3].

One of the principal challenges in clinical endocrine practice is thyroid disease management. During the last years, continuous progress has been experienced in medical science. Also, some factors have improved our knowledge of this field from arithmetical to geometrical proportions. Some of the lists of these factors include accurate clinical assessment, understanding inter or intracellular reactions, and the environment's influence on this reaction [2]. Most fields of science have undergone a big data revolution. The use of data science in personalized medicine is important for treating variability in autoimmune disorders, especially in patients with the presence of varying autoimmune diseases [4, 5]. Studies have also shown how data like the electronic health records (EHRs) initially designed to facilitate patients registration has been used as a tool in predicting thyroid diseases, as seen in some reports that link the EHRs data to extant genotypes to identify new gene locus like forkhead box E1 (FOXE1), which is associated with autoimmune thyroid diseases [6–8].

Genomic data is an important data in precision medicine. Therefore, most thyroid diseases such as autoimmune thyroiditis are known to have high heritability [8, 9]. Studies have reported high rate of Graves' disease in monozygotic twins compared to dizygotic twins (in the range of 50–70%, compared with 3–25% respectively). Also, Hemminki and his co-worker reported the familial standardized incidence ratios for Graves' disease to be 4.49 (for individuals whose parent was affected), 5.04 (for individuals with only a single sibling affected), while 310 (if the individual has two or more siblings affected), and 16.45 in twins [1, 8, 10]. For Hashimoto's thyroiditis (HT), the sibling risk ratio was found to be 28 and this risk was confirmed in data obtained from Germany [8, 11, 12]. All this evidence shows the association of genetic susceptibility to autoimmune thyroid diseases.

A genome-wide association study (GWAS) of hyperthyroidism was carried out with a sample of 1317 hypothyroidism cases and 5053 controls which was algorithmically determined from five EMRDs (electronic medical record databases), one association was found with near forkhead box E1 (also known as thyroid transcription factor 2 (TTF-2)) [7]. Gene studies have also linked autoimmune hypothyroidism with PTPN22 (protein tyrosine phosphatase, non-receptor type 22), CTLA4 (cytotoxic T lymphocyte antigen 4) and HLA II (human leukocyte antigen class II region) [7, 8]. On the other hand, Graves' disease has been studied in several genome-wide association studies, with the discovery of many loci [1, 7]. These associations are important in the diagnosis and treatment of autoimmune thyroid diseases.

2. Autoimmune thyroid diseases and data science

2.1 Autoimmune thyroid diseases (AITDs)

Autoimmune thyroid diseases (AITDs) are the most common autoimmune diseases in humans and it is divided based on the grade of lymphocytic infiltration [13]. They are more prevalent in females than males (i.e. they are 5–10 less frequent in men). Graves' disease which is a disease associated with hyperthyroidism and Hashimoto's thyroiditis which is also associated with hypothyroidism are the major types of AITDs [13].

2.1.1 Graves diseases (GD)

Graves' disease is the most common cause of hyperthyroidism, which affects people at any age but most prevalent in adults, the incidence of this disease peaks between 30 and 50 years [14]. It is also characterized by goiter, ophthalmopathy [15].

2.1.2 Hashimoto's thyroiditis (HT)

HT has now been considered the most common AITD [16], the most common endocrine disorder [17] and also the most common cause of hypothyroidism [18, 19]. It can be divided into primary and secondary forms, the primary form is the most common thyroiditis and the secondary is the more recent description of thyroiditis [20].

2.2 Causes of AITDs

The factors that result in AITDs are genetic factors and environmental factors. Various susceptibility genes like HLA-DR gene locus and non-MHC genes which includes CTLA-4, CD40, PTPN22, CD25, FOXP3, thyroglobulin and TSH receptor genes have been identified and characterized [21]. The major environmental triggers that have been identified are; iodine, selenium, medications, smoking and stress, infection, sex steroids, pregnancy, fetal microchimerism and radiation exposure [22, 23].

The risk of developing Graves' disease is influenced by genetic factors accounting for up to 80%, while environmental factors account for up to 20% [24–26]. The mechanisms involved in immune tolerance are destroyed by these environmental factors in genetically predisposed people leading to the onset of the disease [24, 26].

In Hashimoto thyroiditis, genetic and environmental factors also contribute to the development of HT.

2.3 Pathogenesis of AITDs

Many factors play a role in the pathogenesis of AITDs, mostly involving the complex interaction of the genetics and environmental factors, immune system and cytokines [27]. The pathogenesis of AITDs results from either cell-mediated autoimmune and endocrine autoimmunity [26]. Thyroid peroxidase antibodies are potent marker of AITDs [27]. Its levels associated with the expression of MHC on thrococytes and with a degree of infiltration by lymphocytes may sensitize and trigger the synthesis of autoantibodies [28]. They are involved in both the immune system and directly targeting the thyroid follicular cells [27]. Their presence has been identified within inflammatory and thyroid follicular cells [29]. Cytokines enhance inflammatory responses by stimulating both B and T lymphocytes, resulting in antibody production and damage to the thyroid tissue by apoptosis in particular HT [30]. In addition, T cells subtypes have also been recently discovered to play a role in the pathogenesis of AITDs [31–33].

In Graves' disease, pathogenesis is a complex process, it involves the TRAbs which are antibodies against the thyroid-stimulating receptors [34]. TSH receptor antibodies (TRAb) mimics the function of TSH and it causes the disease by binding to the TSH receptor thereby stimulating or inhibiting thyroid cells in producing thyroid hormones (T3 and T4) [35]. The TRAbs binding to the TSH receptors leads to continuous and uncontrolled thyroid stimulation associated with the synthesis of thyroid hormone in excess and thyroid hypertrophy [35].

In Hashimoto thyroiditis, the pathogenic mechanism involves the contribution of cellular immunity in the form of the defect in the suppressor T cells as well as regulatory T cells, follicular helper T cells, cytotoxicity and apoptosis and humoral immunity in the form of TPO/TG antibodies and immunoglobin subclass, sodium iodide symporter (NIS) and pendrin antibodies, thyroid-stimulating hormone receptor (TSHR) antibodies and also the role of cytokines and DNA fragments and micro RNA [36]. All these have been observed to play an important role in the pathogenesis of HT.S.

2.4 Management of AITDs

The recent landmark in the management of HT disease and GD disease will be discussed as it is the major form of AITDs.

2.4.1 Hashimoto's thyroiditis

Since it discovery, various understanding has been made about this condition. It has been reviewed that a grading system might be a better method of classifying hypothyroidism due to the continuous change that is observed in the serum level of TSH and free thyroxine (T4) than differentiating it into clinical and subclinical forms [37]. With this consideration, it becomes difficult to determine a starting point for thyroid hormone therapy supplementation which is ideal enough. A randomized trial (TRUST) initiated by the European Commission (2012) aids the understanding of the effects of levothyroxine (LT4) in the treatment of subclinical hypothyroidism [37].

Reoccurrence of symptoms was observed in 5–10% of patients with hypothyroidism despite receiving LT4 treatment and having a normal serum TSH levels [38]. A guideline has been provided by European Thyroid Association (ETA) on the combination therapy of LT4 and LT3 as superior to T4monotherapy and LT4 mono-therapy [38].

2.4.2 Graves's diseases

Since the inception of GD, it has been treated by antithyroid drugs, radioactive iodine and surgery. Preexisting guidelines were used in the management of GD but recently a detailed guideline has been provided separately for subclinical hyperthyroidism, although they are not supported by randomized clinical trial [39]. Radioiodine is used in the treatment of Grave's disease [40]. It connects to thyroid autoimmunity through thyroid cell death in which self-antigens are liberated from the thyroid gland following the exposure to the therapy until complete ablation has been achieved [40]. Treatments of GD with antithyroid drugs gives favorable and unfavorable response in patients [40].

With all the recent studies on the management of GD, each management plan is associated with its limitation and a definite plan for the management of GD has not been confirmed. To provide a permanent treatment plan for the disease, researchers are: looking at the aspects of creating a new drug that will d preventing the disease without destroying or removing the thyroid gland and also avoiding the recurrence of the disease. The results of recent in vivo experiments are quite promising [41].

In both diseases, vitamin D has been reviewed to play a significant role in the modulation of the immune system, enhancing the innate immune response while it also exerts an inhibitory action on the adaptive immune system [42].

2.5 General investigation of AITDs

This is based on clinical features and laboratory investigation. The circulating antibodies is a core determinant of AITDs as they are measured against TPO and TG. A negative test excludes AITDs, but a positive test infers AITDs, each type of disease depending on the presence of either antibody. The measurement is done using thyroid receptors assays or bioassays [37].

2.6 Data science approaches to investigate autoimmune diseases

At a time when computer processing power keeps increasing exponentially while networks keep expanding, data available at the same time becomes overwhelming and it becomes imperative to marry the field of data processing and computer so as to take full advantage of the available data as it already exceeds the processing capacity of manual methods and conventional database approach [43]. Data science as a field supports the process of taking data-driven decisions while depending largely on "Big data" storage, engineering and analysis [43]. Therefore thinking data science application in a field implies the intention to gather data, process such data, analyze and utilize such data for the purpose of understanding illness, understanding the reason for such illness (diagnosis), understanding how the illness is progressing (prognosis), understanding the possible endpoint of such illness (prediction) and understanding the intervention that could bring the best out of such situation (treatment/recommendation) [44].

Autoimmune diseases are dangerous or disruptive disease conditions that affect the tissues of the body, which is facilitated by the susceptible genes present in the host and environmental factors where the body's immune system attacks itself through the presentation and recognition of specific antigens and the response of the target organs [45].

2.6.1 Data science approaches

In an attempt to harness the recent and innovative development taking place with regards to computing infrastructure, methods of data processing and tools for data analysis, the discipline of data science is evolving with serious evolving challenges. Cluster computing and cloud computing are fundamental components of data science that enhance usage of powerful algorithms necessary to access, visualize, interpret, organize, analyze, and rapidly with a reasonable degree of efficiency manage cross-scale big data necessary for enhanced use of artificial intelligence. The availability of big data and the advancement in the field of artificial intelligence has led to the development of various machine learning algorithms, deep learning algorithms and deep neural networks algorithms to process big data considering its high volume and complexity.

2.6.2 Machine learning

One big question that has been raised in the field of computing is the question of how to design and enable computers that are capable of improving automatically through the various experience without explicit instructions and limited human intervention. Such question was answered by the birth of the field of machine learning which stands as one of the most rapidly growing technical fields today which is a point where computer science intersects with statistics and stands as the heart of artificial intelligence and data science [46]. The mechanism of machine learning, a rapidly developing arm of computational algorithms, is to simulate and emulate human reasoning and intelligence by allowing the designed system to learn from the environment. Low cost of computation, online access and availability of data, discovery of new theories and new learning algorithms among other are forces that drives machine learning [46]. Different machine-learning algorithms has been made with the intention to solve various machine learning related problems and use the large variety of data types [47, 48]. Conceptually, what machine-learning algorithms do can be perceived as running through a large selection of the program to select a program of choice and this choice is guided by experience acquired through training and the choice would be a program that optimizes the performance metric. The great range of variation seen in machine-learning algorithms depends in part on the method by which the algorithm represents its candidate programs (e.g., mathematical functions, decision trees, and general programming languages) [47]. The variation is also dependent on the method through which such algorithm search through this list of programs (e.g., optimization algorithms with well-understood convergence guarantees and evolutionary search methods that evaluate successive generations of randomly mutated programs) [47]. Supervised learning stands as the most widely employed method of training machine learning algorithms [47].

2.6.3 Deep learning

Deep learning involves the use of computational models that are made up of multiple layers of processing, which are capable of learning using representations of data with multiple levels of abstraction. Deep learning methods have rapidly and progressively improved technologies available for recognizing and processing speech, recognizing and identifying visual objects, and many other domains. Deep learning has also been useful in fields such as drug discovery and genomics. Conventional machine-learning techniques were limited in their ability to process natural data in their raw form. However, deep learning using multiple levels of abstraction and representation that is obtained by making simple but non-linear modules that can transform the representation at one level (starting with the raw input) into a representation at a higher, slightly more abstract level and with the composition of enough of such transformations, very complex functions can be learned [49].

2.6.4 Deep neural network

Multiple levels of non-linearity in the networks of artificial neurons that makes up deep multi-layer neural networks enables such algorithm to compactly represent functions which are non-linear and highly-varying. Some interesting characteristics of neural network-based systems include the fact that they can learn and adapt while learning because they consist of an architecture of artificial neurons which are wired to form networks that are arranged in layers, has a loss or optimisation function driving the learning process and possess a training algorithm constantly run through changing parameters [50].

3. Application of data science in the treatment of autoimmune thyroid diseases

Data science is known to encompass the preparation of data for analysis, this includes aggregating, cleaning, and manipulating the data to uncover patterns and draw out insights. Exploiting historical clinical datasets to improve future treatment choices has proved beneficial for both patients and physicians [43, 51]. Through machine learning (a branch of artificial intelligence), it is very possible to obtain patterns within patient data, the exploitation of these patterns helps to predict and treat patients in order to improve clinical disease management [52].

Machine learning also features selection algorithms such as Kruskal-Wallis' analysis, Fisher's discriminant ratio, and Relief-F. In some research, these algorithms have been used to analyze databases containing clinical features (such as U.S. Surveillance Epidemiology and End Results (SEER) database) from identified thyroid disease patients [51].

Also, the discovery of data mining has been essential in the health care sector as its application have been reported in drug delivery, disease predictions and abnormality detections. Electronic health records have provided access to vast clinical data, the application of data mining techniques has helped transform this data information into valuable knowledge for making health care decisions [53]. Also, data mining algorithms have been used on health record data sets to analyze factors contributing to autoimmune diseases such as those associated with thyroid disease [54].

Although the major autoimmune thyroid disease include Graves' disease and Hashimoto's thyroiditis [55], these diseases are different clinically. Genetic data shows that their pathogenesis shares immuno-genetic mechanisms. Some shared susceptibility genes include human leukocyte antigen DR containing arginine at position (β74 HLA-DRβ1-Arg74). Exploring the genetic-epigenetic interactions of autoimmune thyroid pathogenesis is essential to uncover new therapeutic targets [55], this suggests how important genetic datasets are in developing therapeutic targets.

Precision medicine has also been implemented in a therapeutic approach to autoimmune thyroid disease such as Graves' disease [1]. Therefore, recent therapies are targeting a key co-stimulatory molecule usually expressed on antigen-presenting

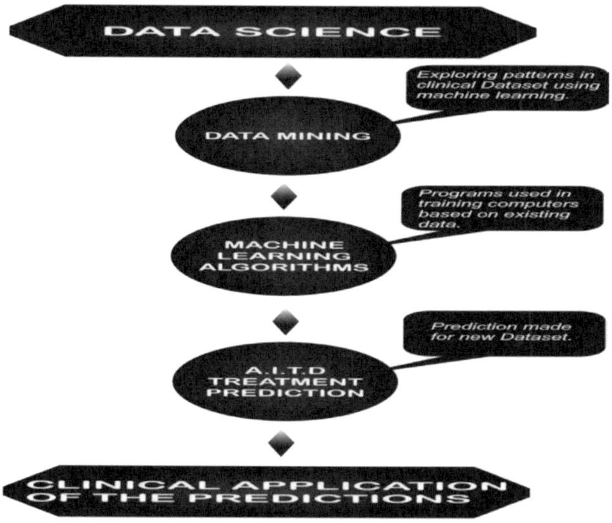
DATA SCIENCE
Exploring patterns in clinical Dataset using machine learning.
DATA MINING
Programs used in training computers based on existing data.
MACHINE LEARNING ALGORITHMS
Prediction made for new Dataset.
A.I.T.D TREATMENT PREDICTION
CLINICAL APPLICATION OF THE PREDICTIONS

Figure 1.
Shows the steps taken in applying data science to treat autoimmune thyroid disease (AITD).

cells (CD40), due to this, anti-CD40 monoclonal antibody has been developed [56]. Studies on genetic data suggest that genetic polymorphisms in the CD40 gene drive its expression and response to anti-CD40 monoclonal antibody like Iscalimab (also known as CFZ 533), which is a full human IGg1 [56, 57]. Furthermore, studies established that thyroglobulin antibody (TgAb) and thyroid peroxidase antibody (TPOAb) are the most characteristic autoimmune antibodies to Hashimoto's thyroiditis [58].

The aim of analyzing datasets (such as genomic datasets and electronic health records) in precision medicine of autoimmune thyroid disease is to determine the treatment options, manner of implementation and choice of therapy. Lastly, this section demonstrate that existing medical datasets has been a reliably strength in clinical predictions, thus, it helps medical practitioners to make an informed and optimized treatment decisions. **Figure 1** illustrates the steps in the application of data science to treat autoimmune thyroid disease.

3.1 Biological agents in treatment of Graves's disease

Biological agents are usually precise for a specified target, a few have subsequently renowned standard target (e.g. rituximab for B-lymphocytes) [59]. Considering specific agents with specific targets is the strategy that aid to achieve cure for this autoimmune disease [60]. Some biological agents involved in novel treatment of Grave's disease include:

a. Rituximab (RTX): rituximab is an anti-B cell agent (monoclonal chimeric antibody) that is against the transmembrane protein CD20 on B cells (but not plasma cells) [61]. Intraorbital administration of rituximab has been shown to be effective as opposed to high dose of systemic glucocorti-coids in the treatment of thyroid-related orbitopathy in grave disease [62, 63].

b. Adalimumab: T-cells expressing IGF-1 receptors are assumed to show a central role in mediating the autoimmune process in severe grave's disease [64]. Adalimumab is one of the anti-T-cell agents which seems to have efficacy similar to that of infliximab. It is a human monoclonal IgG1 antibody which clings to both soluble and membrane-bound TNF (tumor necrosis factor), it also repairs complement and induces lysis of cells expressing membrane-bound TNF [64, 65].

c. Intravenous immunoglobulin: strategically using anti-auto-antigen to stimulate the thyroid but not blocking autoantibodies are highly predominant in severe and vigorous thyroid-associated orbitopathy [66]. Therapeutic measures aiming at the autoantibodies may be effective, even though such consideration must be cross-checked in determining if the presence of such autoantibodies is truly causal or a threat [67].

4. Application of data science in the diagnosis of autoimmune thyroid diseases

4.1 Application of data science in the diagnosis of Graves' disease

The most common cause of autoimmune hyperthyroidism is Graves' disease, which primarily affects the thyroid gland. In Graves' disease, the main auto-antigen is the TSH receptor (thyroid-stimulating hormone receptor (TSHR)), expressed primarily in the thyroid and secondarily in adipocytes, fibroblasts, among others sites. It also appears to be closely related to the insulin-like growth factor 1 (IGF-1) receptor [68]. This disorder presents a systemic clinical manifestation that affect vital organs like the heart, liver and eyes. Failure to diagnose this disease on time can predispose thyroid storm, which carries high morbidity and mortality. Therefore, it is imperative to diagnose and manage the disease early in other to prevent severe cardiac complications such as atrial fibrillation, atrial flutter, and high output cardiac failure [69].

Data mining and machine learning have been reported to play an important role in diagnosing diseases, as they provide a vast classification of accurate techniques for the prediction of disease. Patient data collected from healthcare organizations is useful for accessing the risk factors analysis of diseases such as autoimmune thyroid disease. Classification algorithms is one of the most important applications in the data mining field, which can be used to make decisions in many real-world problems [51, 54]. A recent study uses 34 unique clinical data (variables) such as patients' age at the time of diagnosis and information regarding lymph nodes to build novel classifiers that distinguish patients who probably live for over ten years since diagnosis from those who did not survive at least five years. This report also shows there is 94.5% accuracy in distinguishing patients in terms of prognosis using machine learning [51].

The diagnosis of Graves' disease begins with a thorough historical and physical examination. The historical examination includes the data recorded from family history for Graves' disease, while the physical examination includes assessing goiter size by ultrasound [69, 70]. Dr. Cech began the discussion of precision medicine in the domain of thyroid disease, according to him, the use of radioisotopes to treat hyperthyroidism and thyroid cancer is one of the first uses of precision medicine in thyroid disease [71]. Researchers from the field of endocrine practice investigated Graves' disease retrospectively by collecting data such as disease severity, smoking rate and severity of orbitopathy [70]. Studies have also reported that TSHR antibodies and activated T cells play a major role in the pathogenesis of Graves' orbitopathy, this role is by activating adipocyte TSHR, retroocular fibroblast and IGF-1 receptors, also plays an important role by initiating a retro-orbital inflammatory environment [68].

Since the advent of precision medicine, its future application in thyroid dysfunction suggests developing new approaches in quantifying, detecting, and analyzing biomedical information. Since the description of Graves' disease by Robert Graves, it is known that several environmental and epigenetic factors influence the onset of this disease. Also, some susceptibility elements, such as particular genotypes of HLA, CTLA-4, CD40 or thyroglobulin have been identified. Furthermore, recent data has shed more light on how an epigenetic-genetic interaction between a noncoding single nucleotide polymorphism (SNP) (coded within the TSH receptor (TSHR) gene) alters the thymic expression of TSHR, which further triggers Graves' disease [72–74].

4.2 Application of data science in the diagnosis of Hashimoto's thyroiditis (HT)

Hashimoto's thyroiditis (HT), also known as chronic lymphocytic thyroiditis or chronic autoimmune thyroiditis, is one of the common autoimmune thyroid diseases that can cause an increased tumor vulnerability and raise the chances of developing chronic heart disease diseases especially in individuals with Hashimoto's thyroiditis [75]. The biochemical markers for Hashimoto's thyroiditis are thyroid peroxidase and thyroglobulin autoantibodies in the serum, with greater dominance in females than males. The most significant biochemical etiology of this disease is the presence of thyroid autoantibodies (TAbs) in the patients' serum against two vital thyroid antigens, which are thyroid peroxidase (TPO) and thyroglobulin (TG) [76]. The diagnosis of Hashimoto's thyroiditis (HT) usually causes many controversies, and sometimes until the late stage of occurrence before proper diagnosis can yield result. The use of data science to predict the presence of this dysfunction is key to modern day precision medicine. Firstly, through epidemiological study of the disease pattern in areas where iodine intake is normal or excessive, considering age factor, pathogenesis of autoimmune thyroiditis in monozygotic twins as compared with dizygotic twins [77].

Diagnosis of Hashimoto's thyroiditis (HT) is made by examining a diffuse, smooth, firm goiter in a young woman, with strongly positive titers of TG Ab or TPO Ab and a euthyroid or hypothyroid metabolic condition. This disease caused by immunological damage show conditions that are severe and can cause further complications. Reviewed works of autoimmune hypothyroidism in monozygotic twins, shows there is a corresponding rate below 1 which is traceable to environmental factors and thus, making this factors to be etiologically significant [78]. In precision medicine, the study of genomics can be used to diagnose autoimmune thyroid disease, most especially Hashimoto's thyroiditis. Genotyping analysis to show the genes that are susceptible to environmental factor endocrine disruptors, taking note of the influence of age, weight, sex, timing, and race to show endocrine levels [76].

4.3 Pathogenesis of autoimmune Hashimoto thyroiditis

The presence of TAbs (thyroid autoantibodies) in the patients' sera is the principal biochemical characteristic of HT disease. The Tabs is against two major antigens which are, thyroid peroxidase (TPO) and thyroglobulin (Tg). The TPO antigen is crucial for thyroid hormone synthesis and they are located on thyrocyte's apical membrane, while the Tg are large glycoprotein within the follicular cells of the thyroid gland and they serves as storage for thyroid hormones [76–78].

The principal factor that drives the pathogenesis of HT is the antibodies against TPO (TPOAbs) and Tg (TgAbs) (in immunoglobulin G (IgG) class). Unlike TgAbs, the TPOAbs damage thyroid cells due to its antibody dependent cell cytotoxicity but both shows great affinity for their respective antigens. Furthermore, studies reported that they both have limited role in the pathogenesis of HT but both T-cell cytotoxicity and apoptotic pathway activation influence the disease onset [77, 78]. Although, the TAbs serves as a biomarker for thyroid autoimmunity but TPOAbs are presented in over 90% of HT patients, while 80% of the patients presents TgAbs [77]. Also, T helper cell type 2 (Th2) has been reported to lead to an excessive stimulation of B cells and production of plasmatic cells that produce antibodies against thyroid antigens leading to autoimmune thyroiditis [78].

Table 1 shows some factors that can influence HT [77, 79].

4.4 Importance of data science in thyroid diseases

Studies have reported a vast prediction algorithms that help in classifying, monitoring and suggesting treatment regimen for thyroid diseases, therefore the importance of data science is to serve as early approach to diagnosis, prognosis and treatment of thyroid diseases. Below are studies that achieve a high percentage of accuracy with new data approaches to investigate and treat thyroid diseases.

Since proper interpretation of thyroid functional data is an important issue in the classification of thyroid disease [80], thyroid disease dataset from UCI machine learning database has been used in comparative thyroid disease diagnosis. This was attained by using probabilistic, multilayer and learning vector quantization neural networks [81]. Likewise, Polat et al., also make use of dataset from UCI machine learning repository to diagnose thyroid diseases by hybridizing AIRS (artificial

Genetic factor	A strong genetic susceptibility has been shown to be associated with the disease incidence, development and severity. Of this genes, CTL antigen-4, Tg, vitamin D receptor, cytokines, TPO and PTPN-22 (Protein Thyrosine Phosphatase nonreceptor-type-22) are the most important
Endogenous factor	Most important endogenous factor for this disease are female sex, fetal microchimerism, pregnancy and postpartum period
Environmental factor	Most important factors that influence this disease development are drugs, iodine intake, chemicals/toxins and infections
Self-tolerance	Altered self-tolerance complemented with increased antigen presentation is a strong cause of HT

Table 1.
Factors that initiates Hashimoto thyroiditis.

immune recognition system) which was first proposed by A. Watkins, with developed Fuzzy weighted pre-processing. The classification obtained from this study is about 85% accurate [80].

Moreover, Ruggeri et al., use data recordings of medical history, assessment of selected autoantibodies profiles and physical examination to delineate clinical patterns in patients with Hashimoto thyroiditis from pediatric/adolescent to adult age. It was found out that there is high prevalence of non-thyroidal autoimmune diseases (NTADs) in HT patients and this is also influenced by the patient's age [82]. Therefore, NTADs should be watch out for in patients confirmed to be affected by Hashimoto thyroiditis. Hence, exploring clinical dataset with data science has helped in the prognosis of autoimmune thyroid disease.

Some of the recently proposed algorithms with high accuracy are Expert System for Thyroid Disease Diagnosis (ESTDD), this is an expert system that diagnose thyroid diseases via neuro fuzzy rules with about 95% accuracy [54, 83].

In addition, classification based data mining has also played important role in providing significant diagnosis, decision making and proper treatment for thyroid diseases at early stage. Some data mining algorithms have shown a very high accuracy, speed, performance and low cost for treatments [54]. Example of these

Area	Challenge
Diagnosis	Characterizing the common and individualized genetic background autoimmune thyroid diseases
	Identifying environmental endocrine factors that enhance the development of thyroid diseases
	Predicting the chances of anti-thyroid drug side effects in a particular patient
Treatment	Development of a new thyroid gland from stem cells (for hypothyroid patients (Hashimoto's disease)
	Development of blocking molecules for the self-activated TSH-receptor
	Development of small molecule targeted at thyroid autoantibodies (or gland antigens) to counteract their activity autoimmune thyroid disease
	Precisely tailoring thyroid hormone replacement dose to any patient according to individual needs
	Develop precise targeted immune therapy for the autoimmune disease
	Use of genomic data to predict the chances of acquiring an autoimmune disease in a patient

Table 2.
Challenges in diagnosing and treating autoimmune thyroid disease [68].

algorithms that helps to find better treatments for thyroid patients are kNN (k nearest-neighbor), support vector machine, ID3ara and Naïve bayes [54]. Lastly, novel intelligent hybrid decision support system was utilized in the diagnosis of thyroid disorder, the classification analysis made by algorithms were sensitive, specific and high in accuracy (94.7%, 99.7% and 98.5% respectively). It was also reported that this approach can be applied to other deadly diseases [84].

4.5 Challenges in diagnosing and treating autoimmune thyroid disease

Given the ease of diagnose and treatment of thyroid disease, expectations are high on the specific and personalized approach to the diagnosis and treatment of such disease. However, some aspect of the methods of diagnosis and treatment needs improvement to enhance the health of thyroid disease patients. **Table 2** discusses few of the challenges that has been identified or associated with the management of thyroid related diseases.

5. Conclusion

Data science has been shown to be a useful tool in preparing, aggregating, cleaning, and manipulating clinical data to uncover disease patterns and draw insights into how the disease can be treated. Also, genomic datasets in databases have been utilized in precision medicine to diagnose and treat patients. These facts show green light for data science usage by medical practitioners and researchers in the near future.

6. Recommendations

It is recommended that data science be incorporated into clinical practice to improve precise targeted immune therapy for autoimmune thyroid diseases. Also, it is recommended that more research be carried out using genomic data to further bolster the precision from these data in the diagnosis and treatment of individual patients.

Author details

Ayodeji Folorunsho Ajayi*, Emmanuel Tayo Adebayo,
Iyanuoluwa Oluwadunsi Adebayo, Olubunmi Simeon Oyekunle,
Victor Oluwaseyi Amos, Segun Emmanuel Bamidele
and Goodness Olusayo Olatinwo
Department of Physiology, Ladoke Akintola University of Technology,
Ogbomoso, Oyo State, Nigeria

*Address all correspondence to: aajayi22@lautech.edu.ng

References

[1] Galofré JC, Díez JJ, Cooper DS. Thyroid dysfunction in the era of precision medicine. Endocrinología y Nutrición (English Edition). 2016;**63**(7): 354-363

[2] Tumino D, Grani G, Di Stefano M, Di Mauro M, Scutari M, Rago T, et al. Nodular thyroid disease in the era of precision medicine. Frontiers in Endocrinology. 2020;**10**:907

[3] Ng A, Soo K. Numsense! Data Science for the Layman: No Math Added. Singapore: Annalyn Ng and Kenneth Soo; 2017

[4] Teschendorff AE. Avoiding common pitfalls in machine learning omic data science. Nature Materials. 2018;**18**(5):422-427. DOI: 10.1038/s41563-018-0241-z

[5] Cho JH, Feldman M. Heterogeneity of autoimmune diseases: Pathophysiologic insights from genetics and implications for new therapies. Nature Materials. 2015;**21**:730

[6] Denny JC, Bastarache L, Roden DM. Phenome-wide association studies as a tool to advance precision medicine. Annual Review of Genomics and Human Genetics. 2016;**17**(1):353-373. DOI: 10.1146/annurev-genom-090314-024956

[7] Eriksson N, Tung JY, Kiefer AK, Hinds DA, Francke U, Mountain JL, et al. Novel associations for hypothyroidism include known autoimmune risk loci. PLoS One. 2012;**7**(4):e34442

[8] Hwangbo Y, Park YJ. Genome-wide association studies of autoimmune thyroid diseases, thyroid function, and thyroid cancer. Endocrinology and Metabolism. 2018;**33**(2):175-184

[9] Ajayi A, Adebayo O, Adebayo E. Precision Medicine of Autoimmune Diseases. London: IntechOpen; 2020. DOI: 10.5772/intechopen.95248. Available from: https://www.intechopen.com/online-first/74385

[10] Hemminki K, Li X, Sundquist J, Sundquist K. The epidemiology of Graves' disease: Evidence of a genetic and an environmental contribution. Journal of Autoimmunity. 2010; **34**:J307-J313

[11] Villanueva R, Greenberg DA, Davies TF, Tomer Y. Sibling recurrence risk in autoimmune thyroid disease. Thyroid. 2003;**13**:761-764

[12] Dittmar M, Libich C, Brenzel T, Kahaly GJ. Increased familial clustering of autoimmune thyroid diseases. Hormone and Metabolic Research. 2011;**43**:200-204

[13] Banga JP, Schott M. Autoimmune thyroid diseases. Hormone and Metabolic Research. 2018;**50**:837-839

[14] Zimmermann MB, Boelaert K. Iodine deficiency and thyroid disorders. The Lancet Diabetes and Endocrinology. 2015;**3**:286-295

[15] Bartalena L. Diagnosis and management of Graves disease: A global overview. Nature Reviews. Endocrinology. 2013;**9**(12):724-734. DOI: 10.1038/nrendo.2013.193

[16] McLeod DS, Cooper DS. The incidence and prevalence of thyroid autoimmunity. Endocrine. 2012; **42**:252-265

[17] Golden SH, Robinson KA, Saldanha I, Anton B, Ladenson PW. Clinical review: Prevalence and incidence of endocrine and metabolic disorders in the United States: A comprehensive review. The Journal of Clinical Endocrinology and Metabolism. 2009;**94**:1853-1878

[18] Delemer B, Aubert JP, Nys P, Landron F, Bouee S. An observational study of the initial management of hypothyroidism in France: The ORCHIDEE study. European Journal of Endocrinology. 2012;**167**:817-823

[19] Vanderpump MP. The epidemiology of thyroid disease. British Medical Bulletin. 2011;**99**:39-51

[20] Caturegli P, De Remigis A, Rose NR. Hashimoto thyroiditis: Clinical and diagnostic criteria. Autoimmunity Reviews. 2014;**13**(4-5):391-397. DOI: 10.1016/j.autrev.2014.01.007

[21] Camperio C, Caristi S, Fanelli G, Soligo M, Del Porto P, Piccolella E. Forkhead transcription factor FOXP3 upregulates CD25 expression through cooperation with RelA/NF-kappaB. PLoS One. 2012;7:e48303

[22] Iddah MA, Macharia BN. Autoimmune thyroid disorders. International Scholarly Research Notices. 2013;**2013**:Article ID 509764, 9 p. DOI: 10.1155/2013/509764

[23] Tomer Y, Menconi F. Interferon induced thyroiditis. Best Practice & Research. Clinical Endocrinology & Metabolism. 2009;**23**:703-712

[24] Brand OJ, Gough SCL. Genetics of thyroid autoimmunity and the role of the TSHR. Molecular and Cellular Endocrinology. 2010;**322**:135-143

[25] Morshed SA, Latif R, Davies TF. Delineating the autoimmune mechanisms in Graves' disease. Immunol. Res. 2012;**54**:191-203

[26] Morshed SA, Latif R, Davies TF. Delineating the autoimmune mechanisms in graves' disease. Immunologic Research. 2012;**54**:191-203

[27] Mikoś H, Mikoś M, Obara-Moszyńska M, Niedziela M. The role of the immune system and cytokines involved in the pathogenesis of autoimmune thyroid disease (AITD). Endokrynologia Polska. 2014;**65**(2):150-155. DOI: 10.5603/ EP.2014.0021

[28] Caturegli P. Autoimmune hypophysitis: An underestimated disease in search of its autoantigen(s). The Journal of Clinical Endocrinology and Metabolism. 2007;**92**:2038-2040

[29] Ajjan RA, Weetman AP. Cytokines in thyroid autoimmunity. Autoimmunity. 2003;**36**:351-359

[30] Palazzo FF, Hammond LJ, Goode AW, et al. Death of the autoimmune thyrocyte: Is it pushed or does it jump? Thyroid. 2000;**10**: 561-572

[31] Ramos-Leví AM, Marazuela M. Pathogenesis of thyroid autoimmune disease: The role of cellular mechanisms. Endocrinology and Metabolism. 2016;**31**:379-385. DOI: 10.1016/j.endonu. 2016.04.003

[32] Antonelli A, Ferrari SM, Corrado A, Di Domenicantonio A, Fallahi P. Autoimmunethyroid disorders. Autoimmunity Reviews. 2015; **14**:174-180

[33] Weetman AP. Autoimmune thyroid disease: Propagation and progression. European Journal of Endocrinology. 2003;**148**:1-9

[34] Prabhakar BS, Bahn RS, Smith TJ. Current perspective on the pathogenesis of Graves' disease and ophthalmopathy. Endocrine Reviews. 2003;**24**:802-835

[35] Quadbeck B, Hoermann R, Hahn S, et al. Binding, stimulating and blocking TSH receptor antibodies to the thyrotropin receptor as predictors of relapse of Graves' disease after withdrawal of antithyroid treatment. Hormone and Metabolic Research. 2005;**37**:745-750

[36] Ajjan RA, Weetman AP. The pathogenesis of Hashimoto's thyroiditis: Further developments in our understanding. Hormone and Metabolic Research. 2015;**47**(10):702-710. ISSN: 0018-5043

[37] Hiromatsu Y, Satoh H, Amino N. Hashimoto's thyroiditis: History and future outlook. Hormones (Athens, Greece). 2013;**12**:12-18

[38] Canaris GJ, Manowitz NR, Mayor G, Ridgway EC. The Colorado thyroid disease prevalence study. Archives of Internal Medicine. 2000;**160**:526-534

[39] Biondi B, Bartalena L, Cooper DS, Hegedus L, Laurberg P, Kahaly GJ. The 2015 European Thyroid Association guidelines on diagnosis and treatment of endogenous subclinical hyperthyroidism. European Thyroid Journal. 2015;**4**:149-163

[40] Smith TJ, Hegedüs L. Graves' disease. The New England Journal of Medicine. 2016;**375**(16):1552-1565. DOI: 10.1056/NEJMra1510030

[41] Neumann S, Nir EA, Eliseeva E, Huang W, Marugan J, Xiao J, et al. A selective TSH receptor antagonist inhibits stimulation of thyroid function in female mice. Endocrinology. 2014; **155**:310-314

[42] Kim D. The role of vitamin D in thyroid diseases. International Journal of Molecular Sciences. 2017;**18**(9):1949. DOI: 10.3390/ijms18091949

[43] Provost F, Fawcett T. Data science and its relationship to big data and data-driven decision making. Big Data. 2013;**1**(1):51-59

[44] Van Der Aalst W. Data science in action. In: Process Mining. Berlin, Heidelberg: Springer; 2016. pp. 3-23

[45] Marrack P, Kappler J, Kotzin BL. Autoimmune disease: Why and where it occurs. Nature Medicine. 2001;7(8): 899-905

[46] Jordan MI, Mitchell TM. Machine learning: Trends, perspectives, and prospects. Science. 2015;**349**(6245): 255-260

[47] Hastie T, Tibshirani R, Friedman J. The Elements of Statistical Learning: Data Mining, Inference, and Prediction. Springer, New York, NY: Springer Science & Business Media; 2009. DOI: 10.1007/978-0-387-84858-7

[48] Murphy KP. Machine Learning: A Probabilistic Perspective. Cambridge, Massachusetts, London, England: The MIT Press; 2012

[49] Yan LC, Yoshua B, Geoffrey H. Deep learning. Nature. 2015; **521**(7553):436-444

[50] Durstewitz D, Koppe G, Meyer-Lindenberg A. Deep neural networks in psychiatry. Molecular Psychiatry. 2019;**24**(11):1583-1598

[51] Mourad M, Moubayed S, Dezube A, Mourad Y, Park K, Torreblanca-Zanca A, et al. Machine learning and feature selection applied to SEER data to reliably assess thyroid cancer prognosis. Scientific Reports. 2020;**10**(1):1-11

[52] Stafford IS, Kellermann M, Mossotto E, Beattie RM, MacArthur BD, Ennis S. A systematic review of the applications of artificial intelligence and machine learning in autoimmune diseases. NPJ Digital Medicine. 2020;**3**(1):1-11

[53] Bhattacharya S, Sengupta S. Application of data mining techniques in autoimmune diseases research and treatment. In: Machine Learning and IoT. Boca Raton: CRC Press; 2018. pp. 113-131. DOI: 10.1201/9781351029940

[54] Begum A, Parkavi A. Prediction of thyroid disease using data mining techniques. In: 2019 5th International

Conference on Advanced Computing & Communication Systems (ICACCS). Manhattan, New York, U.S: IEEE; 2019:342-345. DOI: 10.1109/icaccs.2019.8728320

[55] Tomer Y. Mechanisms of autoimmune thyroid diseases: From genetics to epigenetics. Annual Review of Pathology: Mechanisms of Disease. 2014;**9**:147-156

[56] Faustino LC, Kahaly GJ, Frommer L, Concepcion E, Stefan-Lifshitz M, Tomer Y. Precision medicine in Graves' disease: CD40 gene variants predict clinical response to an anti-CD40 monoclonal antibody. Frontiers in Endocrinology. 2021;**12**:642

[57] Kahaly GJ, Stan MN, Frommer L, Gergely P, Colin L, Amer A, et al. A novel anti-Cd40 monoclonal antibody, iscalimab, for control of Graves' hyperthyroidism—A proof-of-concept trial. The Journal of Clinical Endocrinology & Metabolism. 2019;**105**(3):696-704. DOI: 10.1210/clinem/dgz013

[58] Jia X, Zhai T, Zhang JA. Metformin reduces autoimmune antibody levels in patients with Hashimoto's thyroiditis: A systematic review and meta-analysis. Autoimmunity. 2020;53(6):353-361. DOI: 10.1080/08916934.2020.1789969

[59] Gillespie EF, Smith TJ, Douglas RS. Thyroid eye disease: Towards an evidence base for treatment in the 21st century. Current Neurology and Neuroscience Reports. 2012;**12**(3):318-324

[60] Bartley GB, Fatourechi V, Kadrmas EF, Jacobsen SJ, Ilstrup DM, Garrity JA, et al. The incidence of Graves' ophthalmopathy in Olmsted County, Minnesota. American Journal of Ophthalmology. 1995;**120**(4):511-517

[61] Salvi M, Vannucchi G, Currò N, Campi I, Covelli D, Dazzi D, et al. Efficacy of B-cell targeted therapy with rituximab in patients with active moderate to severe Graves' orbitopathy: A randomized controlled study. The Journal of Clinical Endocrinology & Metabolism. 2015;**100**(2):422-431

[62] Salvi M, Vannucchi G, Currò N, Introna M, Rossi S, Bonara P, et al. Small dose of rituximab for graves orbitopathy: New insights into the mechanism of action. Archives of Ophthalmology. 2012;**130**(1):122-124

[63] Briceño CA, Gupta S, Douglas RS. Advances in the management of thyroid eye disease. International Ophthalmology Clinics. 2013;**53**(3):93

[64] McCoy AN, Kim DS, Gillespie EF, Atkins SJ, Smith TJ, Douglas RS. Rituximab (Rituxan) therapy for severe thyroid-associated ophthalmopathy diminishes IGF-1R+ T cells. The Journal of Clinical Endocrinology & Metabolism. 2014;**99**(7):E1294-E1299

[65] Keystone E, Haraoui B. Adalimumab therapy in rheumatoid arthritis. Rheumatic Disease Clinics. 2004;**30**(2):349-364

[66] Kampmann E, Diana T, Kanitz M, Hoppe D, Kahaly GJ. Thyroid stimulating but not blocking autoantibodies are highly prevalent in severe and active thyroid-associated orbitopathy: A prospective study. International Journal of Endocrinology. 2015;**2015**:678194

[67] Kahaly G, Pitz S, Müller-Forell W, Hommel G. Randomized trial of intravenous immunoglobulins versus prednisolone in Graves' ophthalmopathy. Clinical and Experimental Immunology. 1996;**106**(2):197-202

[68] Davies TF, Burch HB. Clinical features and diagnosis of Graves' orbitopathy (ophthalmopathy). In: Post TW editor. 2019. Retrieved on

09/11/2021. Available from: https://www.uptodate.com/contents/clinical-features-and-diagnosis-of-graves-orbitopathy-ophthalmopathy#H17

[69] Pokhrel B, Bhusal K. Graves disease [updated 2020 Jul 21]. In: StatPearls [Internet]. Treasure Island (FL): StatPearls Publishing; 2021. Available from: https://www.ncbi.nlm.nih.gov/books/NBK448195/

[70] Rago T, Cantisani V, Ianni F, Chiovato L, Garberoglio R, Durante C, et al. Thyroid ultrasonography reporting: Consensus of Italian Thyroid Association (AIT), Italian Society of Endocrinology (SIE), Italian Society of Ultrasonography in Medicine and Biology (SIUMB) and Ultrasound Chapter of Italian Society of Medical Radiology (SIRM). Journal of Endocrinological Investigation. 2018;**41**(12):1435-1443

[71] Kahaly GJ, Bartalena L, Hegedüs L, Leenhardt L, Poppe K, Pearce SH. 2018 European Thyroid Association Guideline for the Management of Graves' Hyperthyroidism. European Thyroid Journal. 2018;7(4):167-186

[72] Chiovato L, Magri F. The medical management of Graves disease in the era of precision medicine. Endocrine Practice. 2019;**25**(1):112-114. DOI: 10.4158/ep-2018-0528

[73] Brix TH, Hegedüs L. Twins as a tool for evaluating the influence of genetic susceptibility in thyroid autoimmunity. Annales d'endocrinologie. 2011;**72**:103-107

[74] Ando T, Davies TF. Self-recognition and the role of fetal microchimerism. Best Practice & Research. Clinical Endocrinology & Metabolism. 2004;**18**:197-211. DOI: 10.1016/j.beem.2004.03.002|Medline

[75] Stefan M, Wei C, Lombardi A, Li CW, Concepcion ES, Inabnet WB 3rd, et al. Genetic-epigenetic dysregulation of thymic TSH receptor gene expression triggers thyroid autoimmunity. Proceedings of the National Academy of Sciences of the United States of America. 2014;**111**:12562-12567. DOI: 10.1073/pnas.1408821111

[76] Zaletel K. Determinants of thyroid autoantibody production in Hashimoto's thyroiditis. Expert Review of Clinical Immunology. 2007;**3**:217-223

[77] Zaletel K, Gaberscek S. Hashimotos thyroiditis: From genes to the disease. Current Genomics. 2011;**12**(8):576-588. DOI: 10.2174/138920211798120763

[78] Pyzik A, Grywalska E, Matyjaszek-Matuszek B, Roliński J. Immune disorders in Hashimoto's thyroiditis: What do we know so far? Journal of Immunology Research. 2015;**21**(4);523-528. DOI: 10.1155/2015/979167

[79] Akamizu T, Amino N. Hashimoto's thyroiditis [updated 2017 Jul 17]. In: Feingold KR, Anawalt B, Boyce A, et al., editors. Endotext [Internet]. South Dartmouth (MA): MDText.com, Inc.; 2000 Available from: https://www.ncbi.nlm.nih.gov/books/NBK285557/

[80] Polat K, Şahan S, Güneş S. A novel hybrid method based on artificial immune recognition system (AIRS) with fuzzy weighted pre-processing for thyroid disease diagnosis. Expert Systems with Applications. 2007;**32**(4):1141-1147

[81] Temurtas F. A comparative study on thyroid disease diagnosis using neural networks. Expert Systems with Applications. 2009;**36**(1):944-949

[82] Ruggeri RM, Trimarchi F, Giuffrida G, Certo R, Cama E, Campennì A, et al. Autoimmune comorbidities in Hashimoto's thyroiditis: Different patterns of association in adulthood and childhood/adolescence.

European Journal of Endocrinology. 2017;**176**(2):133-141. DOI: 10.1530/eje-16-0737

[83] Al-muwaffaq I, Bozkus Z. MLTDD: use of machine learning techniques for diagnosis of thyroid gland disorder. Computer Science and Information Technology. 2016;**23**:67-3

[84] Ahmad W, Ahmad A, Lu C, Khoso BA, Huang L. A novel hybrid decision support system for thyroid disease forecasting. Soft Computing. 2018;**22**(16):5377-5383. DOI: 10.1007/s00500-018-3045-9

Chapter 3

Morphology Aspects of Hypothyroidism

Fernando Candanedo-Gonzalez, Javier Rios-Valencia, Dafne Noemi Pacheco-Garcilazo, Wilfredo Valenzuela-Gonzalez and Armando Gamboa-Dominguez

Abstract

Hypothyroidism is a common endocrine disorder resulting of low levels of thyroid circulating hormones. The prevalence in the general population varies between 0.3% and 3.7%. Presents as clinical or subclinical disease based on presence of symptoms and levels of serum TSH and free thyroxine and T4, respectively. Hypothyroidism has numerous etiologies, some of them are originated on the thyroid itself and some others are of extrathyroid origin, with variable manifestations. Classified as primary, secondary, tertiary and peripheral. Thyroid autoimmune disease is the principal cause. A new class of drugs against cancer, like the anti-CTLA-4 and anti-PD-L1/PD1 therapies have been associated with primary or secondary hypothyroidism. Endocrine disorders can be difficult to diagnose based only on morphological features because endocrine manifestations are caused primarily by a hormonal imbalance. Hypothyroidism may have a higher risk of morbidity and mortality. Finally, myxedematous coma is the main complication of terminal stages hypothyroidism.

Keywords: hypothyroidism, epidemiology, pathophysiology, etiology, pathology, anti-CTLA-4 and anti-PD-L1/PD1 therapies, treatment, prognosis, complications

1. Introduction

1.1 Anatomy

The thyroid gland is a butterfly-shaped organ formed by a right and left lobe connected at the midline by a thin structure called isthmus. Located in the neck, the thyroid covers the anterior side of the trachea underneath the larynx at the vertebral levels of C5 to T1 (**Figure 1A**). The average size of a thyroid gland is of 5 cm height and 5 cm wide and it weighs between 20 and 30 grams in adults (**Figure 1B**), being a little more heavy in women. Is a highly vascular organ, receiving blood supply from two main sources, the superior thyroid artery, branch of the external carotid artery irrigates the superior half of the thyroid in more than 95% of the population, the inferior half is irrigated by the inferior thyroid artery that branches from the thyrocervical trunk which is a branch of the subclavian artery. Furthermore, the thyroid gland has extensive lymphatic drainage that involves multiple levels of

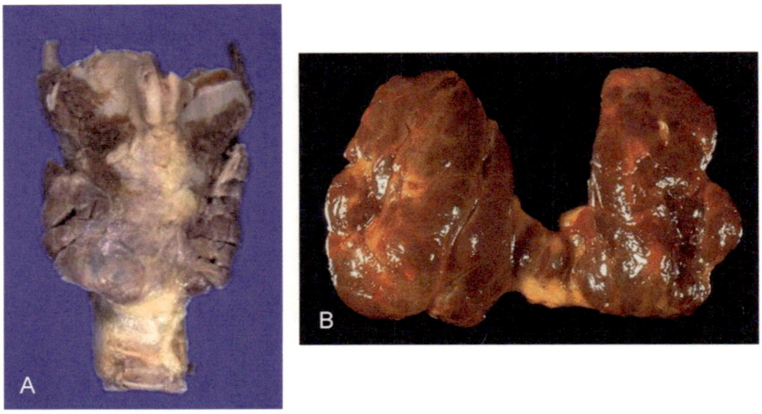

Figure 1.
Thyroid gland: A) butterfly-shaped, located in the anterior side of the trachea underneath the larynx; B) formed by a right and left lobes connected at the midline by a thin structure called isthmus.

lymphatic nodes, including the prelaryngeal, pre and paratracheal, retropharyngeal, retroesophageal and the internal jugular nodes [1].

1.2 Embryology

The thyroid gland is the first endocrine organ that develops during fetal development [2]. It begins to develop during the fourth week of gestation as an epithelial diverticulum arising from the endoderm of the foregut near the base of the primitive tongue, it progressively extending downward starting from week fifth as the fetus develops [2, 3]. It reaches its final shape and size at the end of the seventh week of gestation [2].

1.3 Normal histology

The normal thyroid gland is composed of numerous follicles surrounded by a fibrous capsule that forms septa that divide the parenchyma in multiple lobules. These septa contain nerves and blood vessels that irrigate each lobule. Each lobule

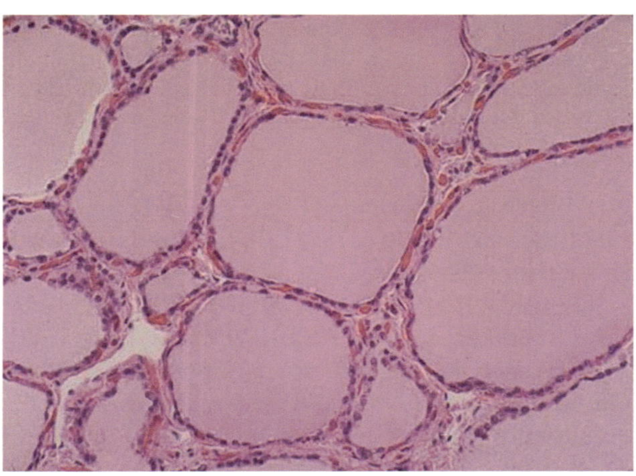

Figure 2.
Normal thyroid gland histology.

contain from 20 to 40 round follicles of 200 μm of diameter on average, these are coated by simple cuboidal epithelium that varies from plane to low according to the current functional activity, when more active the follicle is, taller the follicular epithelium will be. The follicular cells have small, dark and uniform nuclei that are localized at the center of the cell and some of them have an abundant granular and eosinophil cytoplasm, a variant known as Hürthle cells. The follicles contain colloid, a viscous material composed predominantly by the precursor protein of the thyroglobulin (**Figure 2**). The normal thyroid gland contains up to 3 months of thyroglobulin stored in the colloids. Alternating, the parafollicular cells or the C cells, derived from the neural crest through the ultimobranchial body, are found in a higher concentration in the middle and superior portions of the lobes. These cells synthesize and secrete calcitonin, thus participating on calcium homeostasis [4].

2. Definition

Described in 1850, hypothyroidism was the first disorder of endocrine deficiency ever reported [5]. Hypothyroidism is the result of low levels of thyroid circulating hormones. Due to the wide variety of clinical presentations and the lack of specific symptoms, the definition of hypothyroidism is mainly biochemical [6]. Therefore, hormonal levels in overt hypothyroidism are: TSH (Thyroid Stimulating Hormone) >4.8 UI/l, FT4 < 13 pmol/l, and in subclinical hypothyroidism are: TSH >4.8 UI/l, FT4: 13–23 pmol/l [7]. Recent research suggests that the superior reference values for serum TSH varies among different age groups [8]. Nevertheless, up to this present day there is no exact definition of a cut point for serum TSH values regarding age in our population [9–12]. According to the moment of clinical presentation, hypothyroidism is divided in congenital or acquired, according to the level of endocrine dysfunction is divided in primary or secondary or central and according to the severity of hypothyroidism is divided in severe or clinic hypothyroidism or in mild or subclinical hypothyroidism [13].

3. Epidemiology

The prevalence of overt hypothyroidism in the general population varies between 0.3% and 3.7% in the US and between 0.2% and 5.3% in Europe, according to the used definition [6, 10–15]. The National Health and Nutrition Examination Survey found that the prevalence of overt hypothyroidism between people older than 12 years old in the United States is of 0.3% and of subclinical hypothyroidism is of 4.3% [12]. The difference in iodine status affects the prevalence of hypothyroidism, which occurs in population with a relatively high intake of iodine as well as in populations with deficient intake of iodine. The most common cause of thyroid dysfunction is iodine deficiency and it is estimated that 2 thousand millions of people have an insufficient iodine intake [16]. Hypothyroidism is more common in women and the incidence increases with age (>65 years old) and in Caucasian individuals, although data regarding ethnical difference are scarce [6]. Female gender and older age individuals are related to an increase of TSH and prevalence of anti-thyroid antibodies [12]. Among women in reproductive age (12–49 year old), the prevalence of hypothyroidism is of 3.1%. While women older than 80 years old or more, have 5 times more probabilities to suffer from hypothyroidism, compared to the 12–49 year old women population. Hypothyroidism is more frequent among women born with low height and of low body mass index at childhood. However, in countries with good iodine supply, autoimmune disorders are the most common causes of hypothyroidism [12].

3.1 Genetic epidemiology

It is estimated that the heritability of serum levels of TSH and of free thyroxin levels is of 65% and of 23–65% respectively [17, 18]. The results of studies of genome association of all the genome, up to this present day have now explained only but a small proportion of the variability in thyroid function and only three studies have focused on hypothyroidism [19]. The loci that are more consistently implicated in hypothyroidism include genes related to autoimmunity and regulating genes specific to thyroid. The majority of these loci are also related to serum concentrations of TSH within the reference rank [19–23]. Monogenetic disorders that cause congenital hypothyroidism are rare and include TSH resistance (due to an inactivating mutation on the TSH receptor), thyroid digenesis and thyroid dyshormonogenesis.

4. Pathophysiology

To understand better hypothyroidism and its consequences it is important to remember the normal physiology of the thyroid gland. The main function of the thyroid follicular cells is the synthesis of thyroid hormones, tetraiodothyronine or (T4; 3,5,3′,5′-L-tetraiodothyronine) and triiodothyronine (T3; 3,5,3′-L-triiodothyronine). Iodine is essential for thyroid hormone synthesis. Food and water are the main sources for iodine intake, with a daily supply that ranges from 50 to 300 μg being absorbed in the small intestine. Both thyroid hormones are synthesized by the iodination and condensation of two tyrosine molecules and differ by an iodine atom. The production and release of thyroid hormones is stimulated by the hypothalamus-pituitary axis. The thyrotropin-releasing hormone (TRH) released from the hypothalamus stimulates the anterior pituitary gland to release thyrotropin, also called TSH (**Figure 3**) [24]. In response to the stimuli of TSH, the thyroid follicular cells produce thyroglobulin, an inactive protein that is then released from the apical surface into the follicle as a colloid [4]. TSH is released into the bloodstream and it then binds to the thyroid stimulating hormone receptor (TSH-R) in the basolateral surface of the follicular cell of the thyroid gland. The TSH-R is a G-protein coupled receptor and its triggering yields to the activation of the Adenylate Cyclase and of increased levels of intracellular cAMP. An increased cAMP activates the protein kinase A (PKA). PKA phosphorylates different proteins in order to change their functions. The thyroid hormone biosynthesis is made by steps, regulated by enzymes that are stimulated by TSH, these steps are: 1) thyroglobulin synthesis (TG): the thyrocites in the thyroid follicles produce a protein called thyroglobulin. Thyroglobulin does not contain iodine and is a precursor protein storaged in the follicle lumen. Thyroglobulin is produced in the rough endoplasmic reticulum, then the Golgi apparatus packs it up in vesicles and then it enters the follicle lumen by exocytosis. 2) Iodine uptake and transport: the phosphorylation of the kinase A protein increases the activity of the sodium/iodide basolateral symporter protein (Na+/I- symporter), driven by the Na + -K + -ATPase to get iodine out of the bloodstream to the thyrocites. Iodine diffuses from the basolateral surface to the apical surface of the cell, where it transports to the colloid through the pendrin transporter; 3) thyroglobulin iodination: the protein kinase A also phosphorylates and activates the thyroid peroxidase enzyme (TPO). The TPO has three main functions: oxidation, organification and coupling reaction. 4) Oxidation: the TPO uses hydrogen peroxide in order to oxidate iodide (I-) to iodine (I2). NADPH oxidase, an apical enzyme generates hydrogen peroxide for the TPO; 5) Organization: the TPO attaches the remainders of tyrosine from the thyroglobulin with the I2. It generates

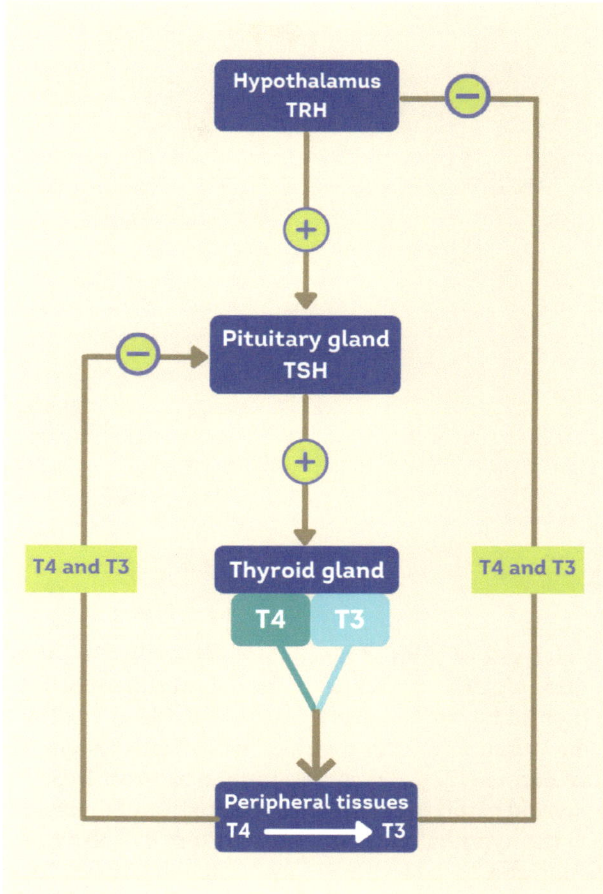

Figure 3.
Normal thyroid physiology.

monoioditytrosine (MIT) and diiodotyrosine (DIT) (**Figure 4**). MIT has only one remaining tyrosine with iodine and DIT has two remaining tyrosine with iodine; 6) mono and diiodotyrosine attachment; the TPO combines the remainers of iodated tyrosine to produce T3 and T4 [4]. MIT and DIT combine to form T3 and two DIT molecules form T4; 5) Storing: thyroid hormones are attached to TG and are storage in the follicular lumen; and 6) secretion: the iodized thyroglobulin returns to the follicular cell, where the degradation of lysosomic proteases releases T3 and T4 in the fenestrated capillaries. Thyroid hormones travel through the bloodstream united to a binding protein called thyroxin [24]. The thyroxine-binding globuline (TBG), transthyretin (TTR) and albumin are proteins capable to bind to the thyroid hormone, thus becoming able to transport it through the bloodstream to their target sites [25].

Thyroid hormones are important for a variety of functions in the body, including development, growth and increase the basal metabolic rate (BMR) affecting circulation, corporal temperature, gluconeogenesis, lipolysis, proteolysis and glucose absorption [26]. It also increases systolic volume and heart rate, which increases cardiac output. In young populations it boosts growth and leads to bony maturation and the fusion of bone growth plates. It is essential for the maturity of the central nervous system (CNS) during fetal development [24]. All of these biochemical events that make the thyroid gland produce hormones is regulated by a negative feedback

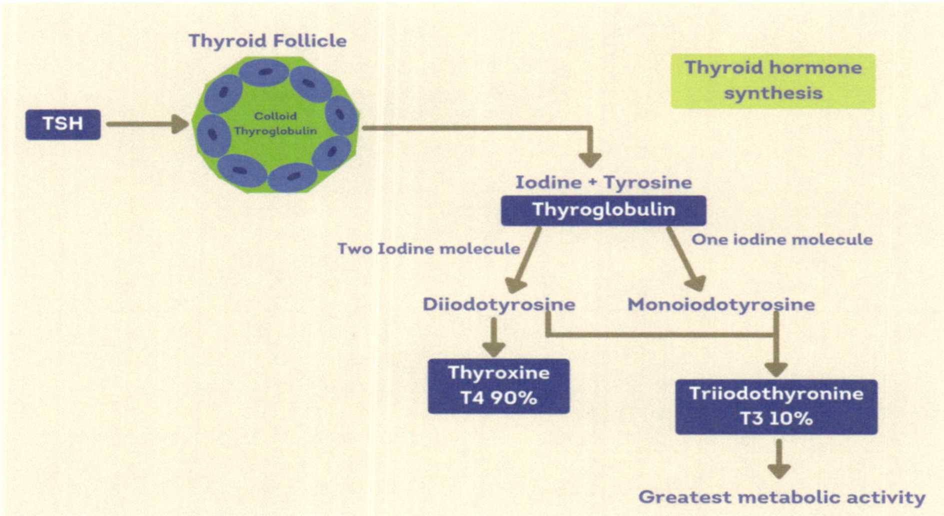

Figure 4.
Thyroid hormone formation.

system in which high levels of thyroid hormones, especially T3, inhibit the release of TSH from the anterior pituitary gland [24]. The counterforces of TRH and T3 allow our body to keep thyroid hormones levels relatively stable in healthy individuals [24]. Although, when alterations occur within this delicate system, severe and even fatal conditions can happen [27]. The most common cause of hypothyroidism is the incapacity of the thyroid gland to produce enough thyroid hormones, nevertheless, with less frequency the hypothalamus and the pituitary can also cause thyroid dysfunction. The half-life of a T4 molecule ranges from 6 to 12 days, in regards to T3 its half-life is of 24 hours, therefore, T4 is significantly more abundant (approximately 100–125 nmol/day) and T3 is found in less quantity, nevertheless T3 is two to tenfold more bioactive [4, 24], to counteract this difference target tissues contain 5′-iodinase, which converts T4 into T3 peripherally through deiodination 5′ [4]. The levels of T3 and T4, mostly T3, establish a negative feedback on the production of TRH and TSH. Alterations on the structure and function of any of these organs or axis can result in hypothyroidism. A decline in the production of T4 results in an increased secretion of TSH by the pituitary, which in turn causes hypertrophy and hyperplasia of the thyroid parenchyma, thus leading to an increase in the production of T3 [4].

5. Etiology

Hypothyroidism has numerous etiologies, some of them are originated on the thyroid itself and some others are of extrathyroid origin, with variable manifestations. **Table 1** resumes the principal causes of hypothyroidism. Hypothyroidism can be classified on primary hypothyroidism, secondary (central), tertiary and peripheral. Primary hypothyroidism occurs when the thyroid gland is unable to produce adequate amounts of thyroid hormones. Secondary hypothyroidism occurs when the function of the thyroid gland is normal and the pathology is on the pituitary gland due to a deficiency of TSH. In tertiary hypothyroidism, the pathology is found in the hypothalamus, due to a deficiency of TRH. Central hypothyroidism (secondary and tertiary) and peripheral hypothyroidism are less frequent and represent less than 1% of all cases [28].

1. Primary hypothyroidism	2. Secondary hypothyroidism	3. Tertiary hypothyroidism	4. Euthyroid disease syndrome
a. Biosynthetic defects:	a. Pituitary destruction	a. Hypothalamic destruction	
Innate errors of metabolism			
b. Development abnormalities	i. Neoplasms	i. Neoplasms	
c. Thyroid destruction	ii. Infarct	ii. Granuloma	
ii. Radiation	b. Isolated deficiency of TSH		
iii. Autoimmune thyroiditis			
d. Thyroid tissue replacement			
i. Neoplasms			
ii. Fibrosis			
e. Drug interference in the production and/or secretion of hormones			

Table 1.
Hypothyroidism causes.

5.1 Primary hypothyroidism

Thyroid autoimmune disease is the principal cause of primary hypothyroidism in the United States and in the geographical regions with enough iodine intake [10]. Hashimoto's thyroiditis (HT) is the most frequent etiology in the United States and has a strong association with the development of malignant neoplasms like papillary thyroid carcinoma (PTC) and lymphoma [29].

There are other causes of hypothyroidism induced by drugs, like amiodarone, thalidomide, tyrosine kinase inhibitors (sunitinib, imatinib), staduvine, interpheron, rifampicin, ethionamide, phenobarbital, phenytoin, carbamazepine, interleukin-2 and lithium. Therapy with radioactive iodine, thyroid surgery and radiotherapy to the head and neck area may be causes of hypothyroidism. Contrary to the previous, smoking and moderate alcohol consumption are related to a reduced risk of hypothyroidism [10].

Post-partum thyroiditis affects nearly 10% of women and generally occurs between 8 and 20 weeks after birth. Only few women will require hormonal treatment. However, some women have a higher risk of permanent hypothyroidism or recurrent thyroiditis postpartum in future pregnancies. The use of radioactive iodine in the treatment of Graves-Basedow disease generally results in permanent hypothyroidism in approximately 80–90% of patients between 8 and 20 weeks after treatment [10]. Treatment with radiation on the head and neck area can also induce hypothyroidism. A relatively infrequent cause of primary hypothyroidism is sub-acute granulomatous thyroiditis (Quervain's disease), it often arises in middle aged women and it tends to be an auto limited disease. Finally, Down syndrome and Turner syndrome patients have a higher risk of hypothyroidism [10].

5.2 Secondary and tertiary hypothyroidism (central)

Secondary and tertiary hypothyroidism, also known as central hypothyroidism, is caused by a defect in the hypothalamus-pituitary axis. Causes include:

pituitary tumors, tumors that compress the hypothalamus, Sheehan syndrome, resistance to TRH, TSH deficiency, lymphocytic hypophysitis, cerebral radiotherapy, drugs like dopamine, prednisone or opioids [10]. A new class of drugs against cancer, like the anti-CTLA-4 (ipilimumab) and anti-PD-L1/PD1 therapies (pembrolizumab and nivolumab) have been associated with primary or secondary hypothyroidism [30, 31]. In previous years, the use of immune check point inhibitors (ICPi) has improved the treatment and prognosis of different types of cancer. The ICPi are monoclonal antibodies associated with adverse effects pertaining the immune system. Thyroid dysfunction (thyrotoxicosis or hypothyroidism) are among the most common adverse consequences. These monoclonal antibodies inhibit immune checkpoints that are present in the surface of the T cells to assure immune auto-tolerance, which results in an increased T cell capacity to attack cancerous cells. The pathogenesis of the thyroid disorders associated to the use of ICPi is not fully understood. Data from observational studies suggest that thyroid dysfunction induced by ICPi is due to a destructive thyroiditis that can evolve to hypothyroidism. On the other hand, it is proposed that thyroid manifestations in patients with immunotherapy may represent an autoimmune phenomenon. Nevertheless, little is known about thyroid antibodies status during the course of the disease [30, 31].

5.3 Peripheral hypothyroidism

Consumptive hypothyroidism is caused by an aberrant expression of the enzyme type 3 iodothyronine deiodinase (D3), which inactive thyroid hormones in tumoral tissues. Even when rare, this overexpression can induce severe hypothyroidism. High concentrations of D3 was first described in a newborn with infantile hepatic hemangioma [32], but it can also occur in patients with vascular tumors and tumors of the gastrointestinal stroma [33].

6. Clinical presentation

Classic signs and symptoms of hypothyroidism are bradycardia, weight gain even when reducing food intake, cold intolerance, dry skin, sweat decrease, constipation, alopecia, hyporeflexia, slow talking and lethargy. Nonetheless, is important to keep high suspicion of hypothyroidism because signs and symptoms can be mild and non-specific. Chronic hypothyroidism also increases total cholesterol and low density lipoprotein and decreases high density lipoproteins, which increases the risk of cardiovascular mortality. Depression is also a common symptom of hypothyroidism and, therefore, it can be found in the medical history of patients that committed suicide [10].

6.1 Subclinical hypothyroidism

A decrease in thyroid function is observed in subclinical hypothyroidism, defined by high levels of TSH and normal levels of free thyroid hormones [34]. Primary hypothyroidism is the most prevalent thyroid dysfunction in elderly population and subclinical hypothyroidism is found nearly in 20% of elderly people [10, 11]. Subclinical thyroid disease during pregnancy can be related to adverse results, including a lower than normal intellectual quotient in the offspring of the pregnant women. It is unknown if the treatment with levothyroxine in women identified with subclinical hypothyroidism or hypothyroxinemia during pregnancy improves cognitive function in their offspring [35].

6.2 Congenital hypothyroidism

Thyroid hormones are extremely important for the correct development of the central nervous system in the fetus. To ensure an adequate availability of thyroid hormones, human chorionic gonadotropin-β (hCG-β) coming from the placenta directly stimulates the maternal thyroid, which increases the production of T3 and T4 during the first trimester. After the first trimester the fetal thyroid converts in the principal source of hormonal thyroid. The placenta also expresses type 3 iodothyronine deiodinase, an enzyme that breaks down T4 into an inverse inactive T3 (rT3), as a protection against excessively high levels of thyroid hormones, however, regardless of this protection, abundant thyroid hormones cross to the fetus [36, 37].

Decreased levels of fetal thyroid hormones during the crucial period of neurologic development drives to severe mental retard, also called cretinism. Therefore, congenital hypothyroidism (CHT) is a pediatric condition that has to be treated with urgency. Other clinical features include musculoskeletal abnormalities, macroglossia and coarse facial features. This condition is irreversible if is not diagnosed early. Even when is not associated to mortality, CHT can be found on fetal and pediatric autopsy for other reasons and must be considered as a differential diagnosis with mental retardation. However, the natural history of CHT has drastically changed in previous years due to newborn screening (NS) programs that consist in detecting this disease in all apparently healthy newborns [36, 37]. In Mexico, the program of NS formally began in 1988 with the emission of the "technical norm 321.4" and in the present its realization is a mandatory action for all health centers that provide child and maternal care, according to the Norma Oficial Mexicana 007-SSA2–1993.5. (Mexican Official Norm 007-SSA2–1993.5) [11, 38].

The main causes that produce CHT are: a) aberrant or incomplete migration of the thyroid bud, which causes the formation of an ectopic gland without lateral lobes, this is also known as a thyroid nodule; b) deficient growth or differentiation that brings about thyroid agenesis or atyriosis, and c) defects on the biosynthesis of thyroid hormones or dyshormonogenesis with or without goiter. The first two entities are grouped under the name of thyroid dysgenesis, which are sporadic and have predominance for the female gender [36–38]. Female predominance is a characteristic particularly interesting in the epidemiology of CHT; although, it is not known if women are more susceptible to develop CHT or if female fetuses with CHT have higher uterine survival compared to masculine fetuses [36]. The molecular mechanisms implicated on thyroid cellular differentiation are not exactly known, yet, some mutations have been described in genes involved in thyroid growth and development, like TTF1, TTF2, PAX8 and TSHR among others [39, 40].

7. Pathology

Endocrine disorders can be difficult to diagnose based only on morphological features because endocrine manifestations are caused primarily by a hormonal imbalance. Nonetheless, anatomical findings, like organomegaly or nodules may suggest anomalies that should encourage further investigation through laboratory tests or microscopic evaluation. Thyroid gland disorders have a wide variety of clinical presentations and can affect many organs and systems.

7.1 Hashimoto's thyroiditis and hypothyroidism

Autoimmune chronic thyroiditis affects from 3 to 5 more times women than men, generally at a median age or older, as well as in children. HT is the most

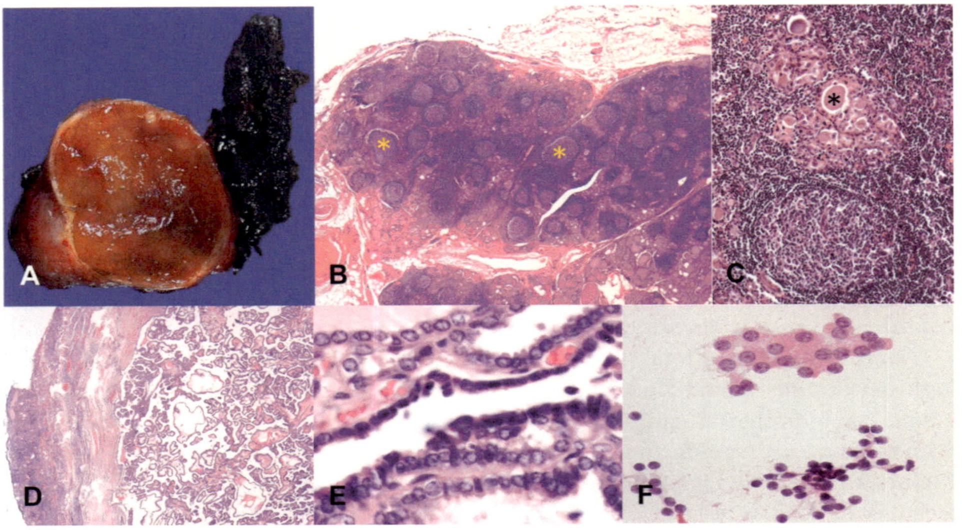

Figure 5.
Thyroid gland: A) product of a hemythyroidectomy with Hashimoto's thyroiditis associated to the presence of a solitary nodule; B) reactive lymphoid infiltrate with lymphoid folliculae with a germinal centers in the thyroid parenchyma (asterisk); C) Hürthle cells (asterisk); D) papillary thyroid carcinoma; E) neoplastic cells with nucleomegaly, open cromatine and nuclear clefts; F) biopsy with fine needle aspiration shows groups of cells with oxyphilic changes (Hürthle cells) and reactive lymphocytes compatible with Hashimoto's thyroiditis.

common autoimmune disease of the thyroid and is the main cause of autoimmune hypothyroidism. This disease was first described by Hakaru Hashimoto in 1912 as a "lymphomatous stroma" [40]. The global occurrence of HT is estimated to be between 0.3 and 1.5 cases for each 1000 individuals per year; predominantly in the female gender; it has a male-female ratio of 5:20 between the 30 and 50 year old population [41, 42]. There are two different clinical variants: the diffuse form and the nodular form. The nodular form is composed by a heterogeneous thyroid parenchyma that presents fibrosis, sclerosis and calcifications and is mainly associated to neoplasms, particularly PTC (**Figure 5A**). It is characterized by a lymphoid infiltrate capable to destroy the gland (**Figure 5B** and **C**), inducing fibrosis and hypothyroidism as a consequence [29]. Chronic inflammation of the thyroid parenchyma is regulated by an infiltrate of predominantly T lymphocytes [13]. The role of autoimmunity is backed by histological findings of diffuse lymphocytic thyroid infiltration and by specific circulating antibodies in almost all patients. Increased levels of anti-TPO antibodies are found in 95% of cases and anti-thyroglobulin antibodies are found in 60% of cases, these being higher in the atrophic form than in the goiter form of the disease [13]. Treatment is almost always non-surgical, surgery is indicated in cases of glandular enlargement with compressive symptoms, non-satisfactory pharmacological treatment and suspicion of neoplasm degeneration in one or more nodules. The association between HT and PTC, first described by Dailey et al. in 1955 [42, 43], is a controversial matter (**Figure 5D** and **E**).

8. Hypothyroidism detection

Even when there are no established guidelines for thyroid disease detection, the American Thyroid Association recommends to start detection at 35 years old and to continue screening each 5 years. Population with high risk of hypothyroidism include: women older than 60 years old, pregnant women, people with a history of head and neck radiation, patients with autoimmune disease, diabetes type 1,

Patients with 4 or more of the following symptoms	Patients with a history of	Pregnant patients with a history of
Fatigue	Sudden and unexplained thyroid growth	Family history of thyroid disease
Sleepiness	Dementia	Thyroid disease during pregnancy
Cold intolerance	Psychiatric diseases	Type 1 diabetes or autoinmune disease
Goiter	Genetic syndromes	
Dry skin	Neck radiation	Complicated pregnancy
Weight gain	Use of drugs that affect	Recurrent miscarriage
Constipation	thyroid function	Menstrual irregularities
	Dermatologic disease	Presence of anti-thyroid
	Hyperlipidemia	peroxidase antibodies
	Cardiovascular diseases	
	Autoimmune disease	
	Hypercholesterolemia	
	Infertility or menstrual	
	irregularities	

Table 2.
Guidelines for plasma TSH measurement and referral to a specialist in cases of hypothyroidism.

positive antibodies against thyroid peroxidase, and people with family history of hypothyroidism [44]. **Table 2** resumes the guidelines for hypothyroidism screening.

9. Treatment

The drug of choice in the treatment of hypothyroidism is the replacement of the thyroid hormones [6, 35, 45].

10. Prognosis

Hypothyroidism may have a higher risk of morbidity and mortality. It can eventually lead to coma or even death. In children, the lack of treatment can provoke severe mental retardation. One of the main causes of death in adults is cardiac failure. With treatment, the majority of patients have a good prognosis and symptoms normally revert within a few weeks or months [46].

10.1 Hypothyroidism complications

Even when is not common, in terminal stages, hypothyroidism, also known as myxedematous coma, is a medical emergency. First described by Sir William Gull in 1873, myxedematous coma has an estimated incidence of 0.22 per million per year [46]. It affects more frequently women older than 60 years old with a large history of hypothyroidism and it tends to occur during cold weather settings. Other triggering factors include infection, cerebrovascular attack, myocardial infarction, traumatism, pregnancy and the use of drugs containing lithium and amiodarone [46].

This affection is associated with a progressive deceleration of physical and mental skills as the disease advances. Initially, symptoms can simulate depression or early dementia, with fatigue, apathy, forgetfulness as the predominant complaints. If not treated, patients can develop severe hypothermia, urinary retention, respiratory depression, bradycardia, hypotension and arrhythmias that include cardiac blocks and torsade de pointes. Torsade de pointes is a non-frequent ventricular tachycardia that is found in a large QT syndrome, caused by an enlargement of the repolarization phase of the action potential. It exists a diffuse deposit of mucopolysaccharides that eventually leads to airway obstruction by affecting tongue and larynx, cardiac tamponade as a result of pericardial effusion and edema without skin and subcutaneous foveae. Electrolyte abnormalities are also produced, specifically hyponatremia and coagulopathies, including the acquired von Willebrand disease, which is associated with an increased mortality [11]. Altered mental state worsens from lethargy to stupor to coma, which increases the risk of aspiration pneumonia, urinary tract infection and sepsis. Mortality in patients with myxedematous coma is estimated to be around 20–25%, which represents a significant improvement respect previous reports of 60–70% due to a better acknowledge and treatment of this disease. Survival rates are worse in elderly patients and in those with severe and or persistent hypothermia, bradycardia, hypotension, lower coma Glasgow score and multiorganic disease. The most common immediate causes of death are sepsis, gastrointestinal hemorrhage secondary to coagulopathy and respiratory insufficiency [10].

11. Directions for future investigation

Even when advances have been made regarding cause detection, knowledge of clinical implications, diagnosis and treatment of hypothyroidism, there are still many questions left without answers regarding diagnosis and treatment. Several risk factors have been identified for abnormal TSH concentrations, concentrations of free thyroxin and thyroid disease, but only a small proportion of these variability is explained. At the moment hypothyroidism diagnosis is based on reference ranks for TSH and free thyroxin. Due to the arbitrary nature of cut points that define mild and overt hypothyroidism, an alternative classification system has been proposed based on thyroid function tests.

Author details

Fernando Candanedo-Gonzalez[1*], Javier Rios-Valencia[1],
Dafne Noemi Pacheco-Garcilazo[2], Wilfredo Valenzuela-Gonzalez[3]
and Armando Gamboa-Dominguez[1,4]

1 Department of Pathology, INCMNSZ, Mexico

2 Student of the Faculty of Medicine, University City, UNAM, Mexico

3 Student of the Faculty of Medicine, Universidad Autonoma de Sinaloa, Mexico

4 Chief of the Department of Pathology, INCMNSZ, Mexico City, Mexico

*Address all correspondence to: fa_candanedo@yahoo.com.mx

References

[1] Beynon ME, Pinneri K. An overview of the thyroid gland and thyroid-related deaths for the forensic pathologist. Academic Forensic Pathology. 2016; **6**(2):217-236

[2] Ozguner G, Sulak O. Size and location of thyroid gland in the fetal period. Surgical and Radiologic Anatomy. 2014;**36**(4):359-367

[3] Takanashi Y, Honkura Y, Rodriguez-Vazquez JF, Murakami G, Kawase T, Katori Y. Pyramidal lobe of the thyroid gland and the thyroglossal duct remnant: A study using human fetal sections. Annals of Anatomy. 2015;**197**:29-37

[4] Mescher AL. Junqueira's basic histology text & atlas. In: Chapter 20, Endocrine Glands. 16th ed. New York: McGraw-Hill Lange; c2021. pp. 348-370

[5] Curling TB. Two cases of absence of the thyroid body, and symmetrical swelling of fat tissue at the sides of the neck, connected with defective cerebral development. Medico-Chirurgical Transactions. 1850;**33**:303-306

[6] Chaker L, Bianco AC, Jonklaas J, Peeters R. Hypothyroidism. Lancet. 2017;**390**:1550-1562

[7] Juárez-Cedillo T, Basurto-Acevedo L, Vega-García S, Sánchez-Rodríguez MA, Retana-Ugalde R, Juárez-Cedillo E, et al. Prevalence of thyroid dysfunction and its impact on cognition in older mexican adults: (SADEM study). Journal of Endocrinological Investigation. 2017;**40**(9):945-952

[8] Garber JR, Cobin RH, Gharib H, Hennessey JV, Klein I, Mechanick JI, et al. Clinical practice guidelines for hypothyroidism in adults: Cosponsored by the American Association of Clinical Endocrinologists and the American Thyroid Association. Thyroid. 2012;**22**(12):1200-1235

[9] Kostoglou-Athanassious I, Ntalles K. Hypothyroidims –new aspects of an old disease. Hippokratia. 2010;**14**(2):82-87

[10] Taylor PN, Albrecht D, Scholz A, Gutierrez-Buey G, Lazarus JH, Dayan CM, et al. Global epidemiology of hyperthyroidism and hypothyroidism. Nature Reviews. Endocrinology. 2018;**14**(5):301-316

[11] Asvold BO, Vatten LJ, BjØro T. Changes in the prevalence of hypothyroidism: The HUNT Study in Norway. European Journal of Endocrinology. 2013;**169**:613-620

[12] Aoki Y, Belin RM, Clickner R, Jeffries R, Philips L, Mahaffrey KR. Serum TSH and total T4 in the United States population and their association with participant characteristics: National Health and Nutrition Examination Survey (NHANES 1999-2002). Thyroid. 2007;**17**:1211-1223

[13] Canaris GJ, Manowitz NR, Mayor G, Ridgway EC. The Colorado thyroid disease prevalence study. Archives of Internal Medicine. 2000;**160**:526-534

[14] Garmendia Madariaga A, Santos Palacios S, Guillén-Grima F, Galofré JC. The incidence and prevalence of thyroid dysfunction in Europe: A meta-analysis. The Journal of Clinical Endocrinology and Metabolism. 2014;**99**:923-931

[15] Hollowell JG, Staehling NW, Flanders WD, Hannon WH, Gunter EW, Spencer CA, et al. Serum TSH, T(4), and thyroid antibodies in the United States population (1988 to 1994): National Health and Nutrition Examination Survey (NHANES III). The Journal of Clinical Endocrinology and Metabolism. 2002;**87**:489-499

[16] Lazarus JH. The importance of iodine in public health. Environmental Geochemistry and Health. 2015; **37**:605-618

[17] Hansen PS, Brix TH, Sorensen TI, Kyvik KO, Hegendüs L. Major genetic influence on the regulation of the pituitary-thyroid axis: A study of healthy Danish twins. The Journal of Clinical Endocrinology and Metabolism. 2004;**89**:1181-1187

[18] Panicker V, Wilson SG, Spector TD, Brown SJ, Falchi M, Richards JB, et al. Heritability of serum TSH, free T4 and free T3 concentrations: A study of a large UK twin cohort. Clinical Endocrinology. 2008;**68**:652-659

[19] Porcu E, Medici M, Pistis G, et al. A meta-analysis of thyroid-related traits reveals novel loci and gender-specific differences in the regulation of thyroid function. PLoS Genetics. 2013; **9**:e1003266

[20] Eriksson N, Tung JY, Kiefer AK, Hinds DA, Francke U, Mountain JL, et al. Novel associations for hypothyroidism include known autoinmune risk loci. PLoS One. 2012;7:e34442

[21] Denny JC, Crawford DC, Ritchie MD, et al. Variants near FOXE1 are associated with hypothyroidism and other thyroid conditions: Using electronic medical records for genome- and phenome-wide studies. American Journal of Human Genetics. 2011;**89**:529-542

[22] Pickrell JK, Berisa T, Liu JZ, Ségurel L, Tung JY, Hinds DA. Detection and interpretation of shared genetic influences on 42 human traits. Nature Genetics. 2016;**48**:709-717

[23] Medici M, Visser WE, Visser TJ, Peeters RP. Genetic determination of the hypothalamic-pituitary-thyroid axis: Where do we stand? Endocrine Reviews. 2015;**36**:214-244

[24] Costanzo LS. Thyroid hormones. In: Cicalese B, editor. Physiology. 4th ed. Philadelphia: Saunders Elsevier; 2010. pp. 401-409

[25] Dai G, Levy O, Carrasco N. Cloning and characterization of the thyroid iodide transporter. Nature. 1996;**379**:458-460

[26] Polikar R, Burger AG, Scherrer U, Nicod P. The thyroid and the heart. Circulation. 1993;**87**(5):1435-1441

[27] Zhang Y, Chang Y, Ryu S, Cho J, Lee WY, Rhee EJ, et al. Thyroid hormones and mortality risk in euthyroid individuals: The Kangbuk Samsung health study. The Journal of Clinical Endocrinology and Metabolism. 2014;**99**(7):2467-2476

[28] Persani L. Clinical review: Central hypothyroidism: Pathogenic, diagnostic, and therapeutic challenges. The Journal of Clinical Endocrinology and Metabolism. 2012;**97**:3068-3078

[29] Graceffa G, Patrone R, Vieni S, Campanella S, Calamia S, Laise I, et al. Association between Hashimoto's thyroiditis and papillary thyroid carcinoma: A retrospective analysis of 305 patients. BMC Endocrine Disorders. 2019;**19**(Suppl. 1):26

[30] Chang LS, Barroso-Sousa R, Tolaney SM, Hodi FS, Kaiser UB, Min L. Endocrine toxicity of cancer immunotherapy targeting immune checkpoints. Endocrine Reviews. 2019;**40**(1):17-65

[31] Sabbagh RE, Azar NS, Eid AA, Azar ST. Thyroid dysfunctions due to immune checkpoint inhibitors: A review. International Journal of General Medicine. 2020;**13**:1003-1009

[32] Huang SA, Tu HM, Harney JW, Venihaki M, Butte AJ, Kozahewich HP,

et al. Severe hypothyroidism caused by type 3 iodothyronine deiodinase in infantile hemangiomas. The New England Journal of Medicine. 2000;**343**:185-189

[33] Dumiltrescu AM, Refetoff S. The syndromes of reduced sensitivity of thyroid hormone. Biochimica et Biophysica Acta. 1830;**2013**:3987-4003

[34] Taylor P, Bianco AC. Urgent need for further research in subclinical hypothyroidism. Nature Reviews Endocrinology. 2019;**15**:503-504

[35] Casey BM, Thom EA, Peaceman AM, Varner MW, Sorokin Y, Hirtz DG, et al. Treatment of subclinical hypothyroidism or hypothyroxinemia in pregnancy. New England Journal of Medicine. 2017;**376**(9):815-825

[36] Vela-Amieva M, Gamboa-Cardiel S, Pérez-Andrade ME, Ortiz-Cortés J, González-Contreras CR, Ortega-Velázquez V. Epidemiología del hipotiroidismo congénito en México. Salud Púb Méx. 2004;**46**(2):141-148

[37] Castilla Peón MF. Congenital hypothyroidism. Boletín Médico del Hospital Infantil de México. 2015;**72**(2):140-148

[38] Flores-Robles CA, Coronado-Zarco IA, Ortega-González C, Arreola Ramírez G, Reyes-Muñoz E. Tamizaje neonatal de hipotiroidismo congénito, análisis de la evidencia actual y propuesta de tamizaje para la población mexicana. Perinatología y Reproducción Humana. 2018;**32**(1):43-52

[39] Di Magliano MP, Di Lauro R, Zannini M. Pax8 has a key role in thyroid cell differentiation. PNAS. 2000;**97**(24):13144-13149

[40] Postiglione MP, Parlato R, Rodriguez-Mallon A, Rosica A, Mithbaokar P, Maresca M, et al. Role of the thyroid-stimulating hormone receptor signaling in development and differentiation of the thyroid gland. PNAS. 2002;**99**(24):15462-15467

[41] Hashimoto H. Zur Kenntniss der lymphomatosen verandererung der schilddrusse strumal lymphomatosa. Arch Klin Chirugie. 1912;**97**:218-248

[42] Dailey ME, Lindsay S, Skahen R. Relation of thyroid neoplasms to Hashimoto's disease of the thyroid gland. Archives of Surgery. 1955; **70**:291-7. 6

[43] Davies L, Welch HG. Increasing incidence of thyroid cancer in United States, 1973-2002. Journal of the American Medical Association. 2006;**295**:2164-2167

[44] Alexander EK, Pearce EN, Brent GA, Brown RS, Chen H, Dosiou C, et al. 2017 Guidelines of the American Thyroid Association for the diagnosis and management of thyroid disease during pregnancy and the postpartum. Thyroid. 2017;**27**(3):315-389

[45] Saudi Arabia and Gulf Thyroid Advisory Board. Protocol for Management of Hypothyroidism: A Consensus of GCC Countries. A Roadmap. London: Springer; 2018

[46] Rodríguez I, Fluiters E, Pérez-Méndez LF, Luna R, Páramoand C, García-Mayor RV. Factors associated with mortality of patients with myxoedemacoma: Prospective study in 11 cases treated in a single institution. The Journal of Endocrinology. 2004;**180**:347-350

Chapter 4

The Role of Ultrasound in Hypothyroidism, Technique, Differential Diagnosis and Follow-Up

Hakan Baş

Abstract

In hypothyroidism, which is as old as humanity, ultrasound has been the first and most important imaging examination in recent decades. This disease is involved in almost all steps in the spectrum from inflammatory diseases to cancer of the thyroid gland. Thyroid ultrasound is a critical tool in the differential diagnosis of hypothyroidism. If thyroid antibodies are negative. It is helpful to determine whether the thyroid is present and to visualize the parenchyma. In a hypothyroid patient, the US may lead to cost savings. If a typical autoimmune pattern is present on US, as a cost-reducing move, further investigations may not be required for the diagnosis of Hashimoto's thyroiditis. Moreover, the ultrasound image may contribute to the decision process whether to treat patients with positive antithyroid antibodies who are euthyroid or have only a mild subclinical hypothyroidism.

Keywords: Hypothyroidism, Ultrasonography, Color Doppler Imaging, Chronic lymphocytic thyroiditis, Thyroiditis, Hashimoto's thyroiditis

1. Introduction

Hypothyroidism that results from low levels of thyroid hormone is one of the most common endocrine disorders. It has various etiology and manifestations; when it is untreated, it increases morbidity and mortality. While the main cause of hypothyroidism is still iodine-deficient diet worldwide, it is autoimmune thyroid disease (also known as Hashimoto's thyroiditis) in regions where dietary iodine intake is sufficient. Today, it is successfully treated with exogenous thyroid hormone [1]. Hypothyroidism often accounts for a large part of the daily practice workload of endocrinology and radiology. Multidisciplinary communication is very important in the approach and management of this endocrine disorder. In the last 30–40 years, the most specific imaging tool in routine examination of thyroid gland diseases is ultrasonography (US). In this section, in hypothyroidism, details about the technique of thyroid US, "pattern recognition", which are important in differential diagnosis, and follow-up will be shared.

2. The thyroid ultrasonography

Ultrasound has become an essential complement to the examination today, while it was used as a new diagnostic tool in thyroid disorders in the 1960s [2]. Ultrasonography has changed the practice of medicine fairly. Relatively easy to use, no ionizing radiation, low cost, and bedside availability have made it invaluable in many clinical settings where patients with thyroid disease are evaluated. The superficial location of the thyroid gland in ultrasonography creates the advantage of high resolution to evaluate thyroid parenchyma and thyroid lesions. US is an indispensable examination in almost the entire spectrum of thyroid diseases. This proposition is similar for hypothyroidism. On the other hand, in thyroid US, specific pattern recognition of the various sonographic presentations of autoimmune diffuse thyroid disease, especially in the clinical presentation of hypothyroidism without antibodies, is completely required. It is also essential in determining whether a focal abnormality represents a true nodule that may require fine-needle aspiration biopsy or is part of an inflammatory process, often referred to as a pseudonodule [3]. The ultrasound, like other tests, should be used to confirm the differential diagnosis when a specific diagnostic question raised by clinical history and physical examination needs to be answered [4]. It should be correlated precisely

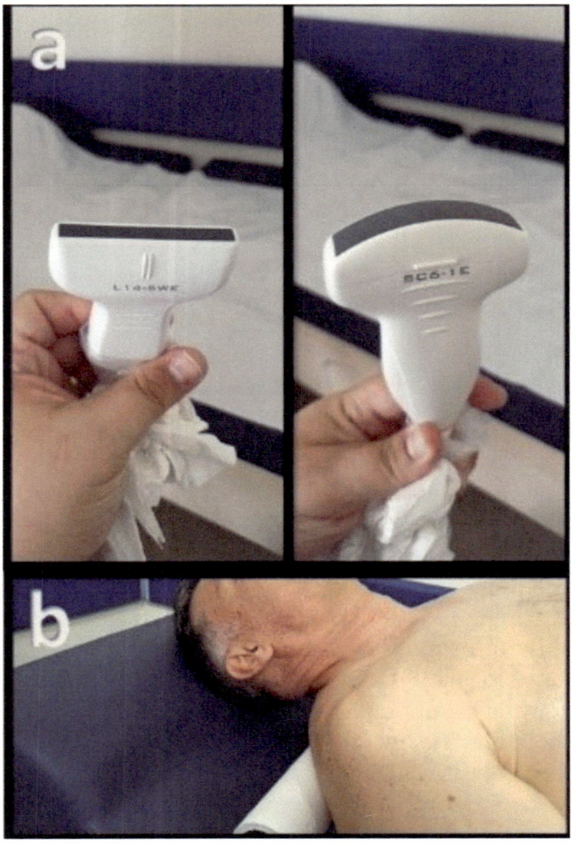

Figure 1.
(a) The lineer and convex transuders. (b) The ideal position of the patient is seen. Procedure is conducted with the patient lying supine with the neck in hyperextension with as much tolerated. Their shoulders can be supported with a rolled towel as seen.

with the other data. The justification of the request for thyroid ultrasound should be made by considering the patient history and laboratory results together.

2.1 The patient preparation, equipments and technique

For the thyroid gland ultrasound, no special preparation is required for the examination. However, the patient is requested to remove jewelry such as necklaces before the procedure. Fasting is not required.

Ultrasound studies of extracranial head and neck structures, including the thyroid gland, should first be performed with a linear transducer. The equipment should be set to utilize at the highest frequency, considering a balance between resolution and tissue penetration. Average frequencies of 7 to 15 MHz or higher are preferred, although some patients may require a lower frequency transducer for deep penetration. In addition, a curved transducer may be necessary to evaluate deep or large structures [5, 6]. The transducers are shown in **Figure 1a**.

The procedure is conducted with the patient lying supine with the neck in hyperextension as much as tolerated. Their shoulders can be supported with a rolled towel so that they can keep their necks comfortably in the hyperextension position [5]. The ideal position of the procedure is seen in **Figure 1b**. Upright or seated

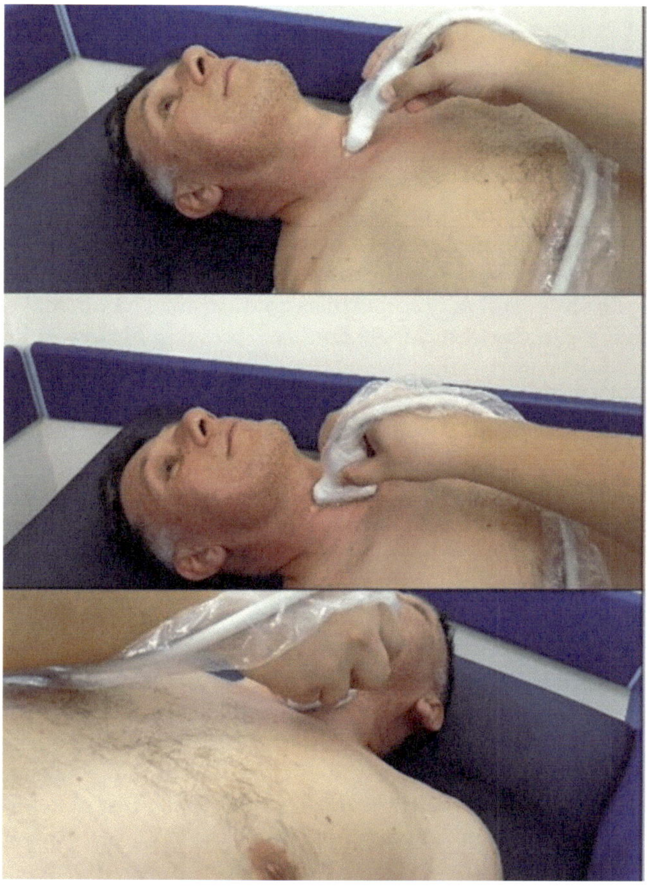

Figure 2.
The examination steps. Firstly, the transducer is perpendicular to the neck long axis for the transverse plane. Then the transducer is turned mild oblique craniocaudally for the sagittal view of right and left lobes, respectively.

positioning may be helpful in patients who cannot tolerate neck hyperextension in the supine position [5, 7].

Water-based ultrasound gel reduces contact loss at the interface between the transducer and skin and improves image quality. It should be applied to the tip of the transducer rather than the patient's neck for patients' comfort. In addition, gel warmers can be used for the elderly and children (especially neonates), where heat loss may have important clinical consequences.

The lobes should be imaged in transverse and longitudinal planes and the isthmus in the transverse plane. Size should be obtained for each lobe, including the anteroposterior, transverse, and sagittal dimensions. In addition, the anteroposterior dimension of the isthmus should be measured in the transverse plane. Color Doppler images are obtained to supplement grayscale images in the appropriate clinical setting [5]. All the examination is illustrated in **Figure 2**. Assessment of the thyroid also includes imaging of the lymph node chain bilaterally for enlarged or abnormal lymph nodes, especially in levels III, IV and VI [6].

2.2 Ultrasound of the normal thyroid

The thyroid is a bilobed gland located anterior to the neck, in front of the trachea, and each lobe is located on either side of the trachea. Both lobes extend vertically and craniocaudally. The isthmus is the part of the gland just anterior of the trachea that connects the two lobes like a bridge. The trachea lies craniocaudal behind the isthmus in the form of an air-filled column. The carotid sheath consisting of the common carotid artery medially and the jugular vein laterally is observed on both posterolateral of the thyroid lobes. Visualized muscles deep in the skin-subcutaneous adipose tissue, sternohyoid, sternothyroid, sternocleidomastoid, and longus colli, also called strap muscles, cover the thyroid gland. The sternohyoid and sternothyroid lie on the anterior of the gland, the sternocleidomastoid lie anterolaterally, and longus colli muscles are located in the posterior of the gland. Another structure that can be seen better in the axial plane is the esophagus, which is located posterior to the left lobe and may sometimes contain air. The normal thyroid sonographic features in the transverse plane are shown in **Figure 3**.

Due to its colloidal content, the normal thyroid gland attenuates more sound beams than the strap muscles, and therefore sonographically appears hyperechoic. Normal thyroid echotexture is defined as uniform and homogeneous hyperechoic. It has a well-defined peripheral margin. In addition, the anterior margin of the thyroid gland is flat or concave. The anterior margin of the normal gland is presented in **Figure 4**.

The normal size of the thyroid gland varies according to the gender and height of the patients. Still, in adults, each lobe is approximately 5 x 2 x 2 cm in sagittal, anterior–posterior and transverse dimensions, respectively. The isthmus is measured in the transverse plane, and its normal size-upper limit is accepted as 0.3 cm. When these dimensions are exceeded, it is understood that the thyroid gland enlarges; this concept is called "goiter". Apart from measurements, some imaging findings can diagnose goiter. The bulge on the anterior surface of the lobes is a clue for diagnoses; as mentioned above, the surface is typically symmetrical and has a flat or concave appearance. The extension of the gland over the anterior surface of the common carotid artery in the transverse plane may be further evidence of gland enlargement. The normal thyroid gland can extend over the carotid surface without enlarging; in this case, the anterior contour shape is important. If it is flat or concave, goiter should not be diagnosed. The group in which the shape and contour of the gland are more important than the size is the children. The gland shape and contour are used to indicate gland growth rather than size [8]. There is no clear

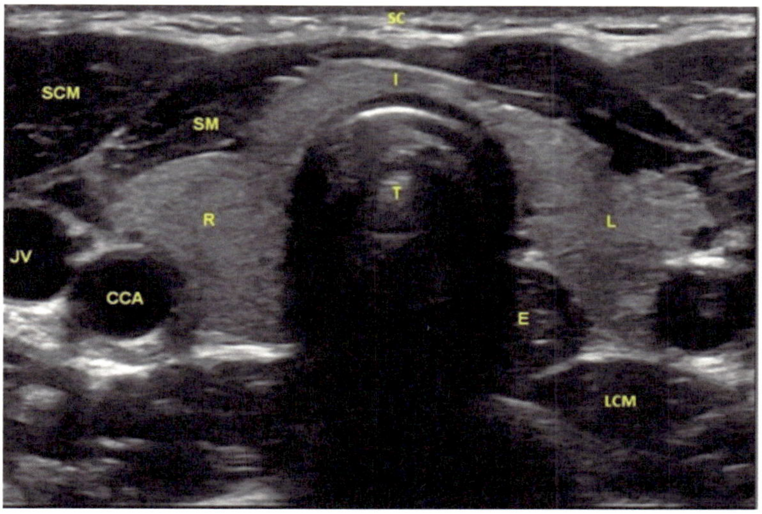

Figure 3.
The normal appearance of the thyroid gland in the ultrasonography examination is presented. (R: right lobe, L: left lobe, I: isthmus, T: trachea, E: esophagus, CCA: common carotid artery, JV: jugular vein, SM: strap muscle, SCM: sternocleidomastoid muscle, LCM: longus colli muscle, SC: subcutaneous tissue).

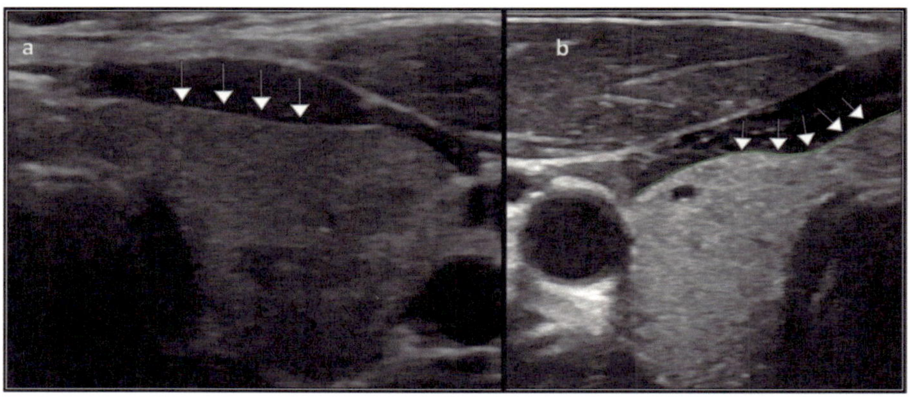

Figure 4.
(a) When the size of the gland is normal, the shape of the anterior surface (arrows) of the gland is nearly flat or (b) concave (green line and arrows). Please pay attention that there is no bulging anterior surface of the gland and no extension of the gland over the anterior surface of the common carotid artery in the transverse plane.

consensus on the normal dimensions of the thyroid in the pediatric population. When calculating the thyroid volume, the ellipsoid formula of width x length x height x 0.523 is used. In epidemiological studies, factors that affect pediatric thyroid size, such as ethnicity and local iodine burden/intake, can be counted [9, 10]. Neonatal thyroid volumes range from 0.84 ± 0.38 mL to 1.62 ± 0.41 mL [11]. The more practical method, the tracheal index, can be used. In the transverse plane, the transverse diameters of both lobes are summed and proportioned to the transverse diameter of the trachea. The normal range of the index is considered to be 1.7–2.4 [12]. Practical measurement methods for goiter are shown in **Figure 5**.

In the normal thyroid gland parenchyma, less than 5 vascular coding is expected in the sampling window at the lowest pulse repetition frequency (PRF) values without background noise on color Doppler ultrasound (CDI).

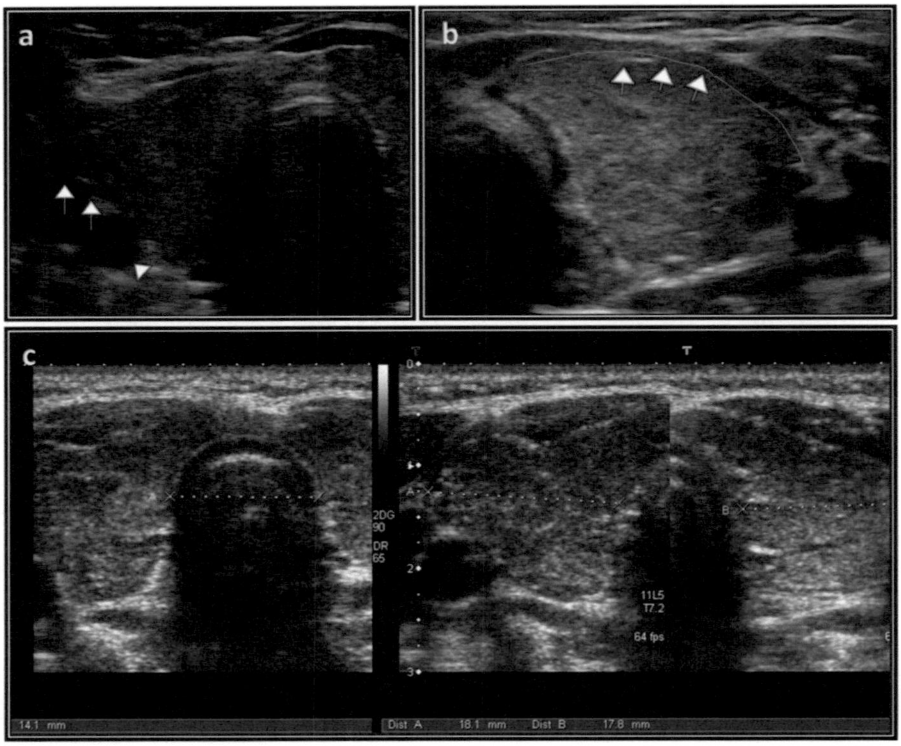

Figure 5.
Practical measurement methods for goiter There is an extension (arrows) of the gland over the anterior surface of the common carotid artery (arrowhead) in the transverse plane (a). The anterior surface (arrows) of the gland is bulging and convex (green line) (b). The right and left lobes dimensions in the transverse plane are 18.1 and 17.8 mm, respectively. The transverse diameter of the trachea is 14.1 mm. In the transverse plane, the transverse diameters of both lobes are summed and divided to the transverse diameter of the trachea. The tracheal index is calculated as 2,45 and interpreted as goiter. Cause normal range of the index is considered to be 1.7–2.4. This method is more appropriate for the pediatric population(c, Courtesy of Prof Dr. Suat Fitoz from his archive. Department of Pediatric Radiology, Ankara University School of Medicine, Ankara/ Turkey).

3. Hypothyroidism

Hypothyroidism that results from low levels of thyroid hormone is one of the most common endocrine disorders. It has various etiology and manifestations; when it is untreated, it increases morbidity and mortality. The etiology of the hypothyrodism is seen in **Table 1**. While the main cause of hypothyroidism is still iodine-deficient diet worldwide, it is autoimmune thyroid disease (also known as Hashimoto's thyroiditis) in regions where dietary iodine intake is sufficient. Today, it is successfully treated with exogenous thyroid hormone [1]. According to the NHANESIII (National Health and Nutrition Examination Survey), based on a population study consisting of 12 years old and older, the prevalence of overt hypothyroidism among adults in the United States was 0.3% and subclinical hypothyroidism 4.3%. Female gender and increasing age were associated with presence of thyroid disorders and abnormality of thyroid lab results [13].

Basically, as related to the region, hypothyroidism etiologies are divided into two categories. If there is a problem with thyroid gland, it is named as "primary hypothyroidism". While the problem with hypothalamic-pitutary axis, it is named as "secondary (or central) hypothyoridism". The role of the ultrasound in

Primary hypothroidism
Fetal hypothyroidism (maternal thyroid-blocking antibodies, maternal antithyroid medication, maternal iodine deficiency, and iodine overload (such as from iodine-based antiseptics))
Congenital hypothyroidism *Transient* (maternal thyroid-blocking antibodies, maternal antithyroid medication, maternal iodine deficiency, and iodine overload (such as from iodine-based antiseptics)) *Permanent* • Thyroid dysgenesis (Agenesis, hemiagenesis, hypoplasia, and ectopia.) • Dyshormonogenesis
Iodine deficiency
Thyroiditis • Chronic lymphocytic thyroiditis (named as Hashimoto thyroiditis) • Subacute granulomatous thyroiditis (named as De Quervain disease) • Painless thyroiditis (Silent thyroiditis-Postpartum thyroiditis) • Suppurative thyroiditis • Drug-induced thyroiditis
Others Surgery, Thyroid radioactive iodine therapy, Radiotherapy to head or neck area
Secondary (central) hypothyroidism Neoplastic, infiltrative, inflammatory, genetic or iatrogenic disorders of the pituitary or hypothalamus.

Table 1.
The etiology of the hypothyrodism.

hypothyroidism reveals, when the etiology is primary hypothyroidism. Patients are usually referred to radiology clinics if elevated thyroid stimulating hormone (TSH) levels or palpable goiter are detected. In addition, also, when incidentally an abnormality is detected in the neck ultrasound, and for control purposes during pregnancy and before pregnancy.

With appropriate clinical history and laboratory results, ultrasonography in hypothyroidism can play an active role in differential diagnosis, follow-up, and treatment decision in some cases. For this reason, interdisciplinary communication should be at the highest level.

4. The role of thyroid ultrasound in hypothyroidism

In this section we will discuss ultrasound about findings, importance and role in differential diagnosis based on etiology of primary hypothyroidism.

4.1 Fetal hypothyroidism

Transplasental migration of maternal thyroid-blocking antibodies, and maternal antithyroid medication to fetus, maternal iodine deficiency on dietary, and iodine overload such as from iodine-based antiseptics can cause fetal hypothyroidism. Similar reasons may lead to transient congenital hypothyroidism in the newborn period after delivery. Fetal hypothyroidism is clinically associated with an increased risk of miscarriage and recurrent miscarriages, prematurity, impaired neurolation, and mental retardation.

In pregnancy, ultrasonography is a helpful tool to assess thyroid status in utero [7]. Ranzini et al. created the nomograms of fetal thyroid size by using the 5th, 10th, 50th, 90th, and 95th percentiles based on biparietal diameter and gestational age. They measured thyroid circumference without intraobserver or interobserver variability. It was found that variations in thyroid circumference measurements increased with both larger biparietal diameter and advancing gestational age. The context of this study is that fetal goiter may develop during pregnancy in women with Graves' disease and taking antithyroid drugs. Evaluation of goiter in the fetuses of these patients is important in terms of justifying the invasive and risky procedures such as amniocentesis, which is necessary for the determination of fetal thyroid hormone status [14]. In some case reports, fetal goiter and hypothyroidism have been investigated and it has been reported that it can be successfully treated with intraamniotic injections of tri-iodothyronine and thyroxine. It is thought that recognition and treatment of fetal goiter can reduce obstetric complications and improve the prognosis for normal growth and mental development of affected fetuses [15, 16]. Evaluation of fetal thyroid size in mothers with Graves' disease may also be useful in adjusting the dose of antithyroid medication and preventing fetal and neonatal goiter and hypothyroidism [7].

4.2 Congenital hypothyroidism

The incidence of congenital hypothyroidism is 1 in 1,400–4,000 newborns. Early diagnosis of hypothyroidism is very important by screening with the Guthrie test performed on the 5th postnatal day. After an abnormal Guthrie test, it is necessary to investigate the etiology and start hormone replacement therapy quickly to ensure proper neuronal and psychological growth [11]. Congenital hypothyroidism can be divided into two major categories: transient and permanent.

4.2.1 Transient congenital hypothyroidism

Transplacental migration of maternal thyroid-blocking antibodies and maternal antithyroid medication to the fetus, maternal iodine deficiency on dietary, and iodine overload such as from iodine-based antiseptics can cause transient congenital hypothyroidism in the newborn period after delivery. Newborns with transient congenital hypothyroidism do not need lifelong replacement therapy. Since this situation is temporary, no further imaging is required [17].

4.2.2 Permanent congenital hypothyroidism

Causes of permanent congenital hypothyroidism include thyroid dysgenesis responsible for about 80% of cases, dyshormonogenesis responsible for about 20%, and rarely seen hypopituitarism (not mentioned here). In congenital hypothyroidism, US examination is the primary method for distinguishing orthotopic from ectopic thyroid; then, further investigation is thyroid scintigraphy.

4.2.2.1 Thyroid dysgenesis

Athyreosis refers to an empty thyroid lodge caused by agenesis or ectopia and manifests as an empty fossa. In the presence of athyreosis, the presence of echogenic triangles, usually smaller than 5 mm, on both sides of the trachea, representing ultimobranchial and connective tissue residue, maybe misinterpreted as hypoplastic or dysplastic thyroid. This tissue, sometimes containing microcysts, does not flow or is minimal on color Doppler examination [18, 19]. The ultrasound finding of the athyreosis caused by agenesia is seen in **Figure 6**.

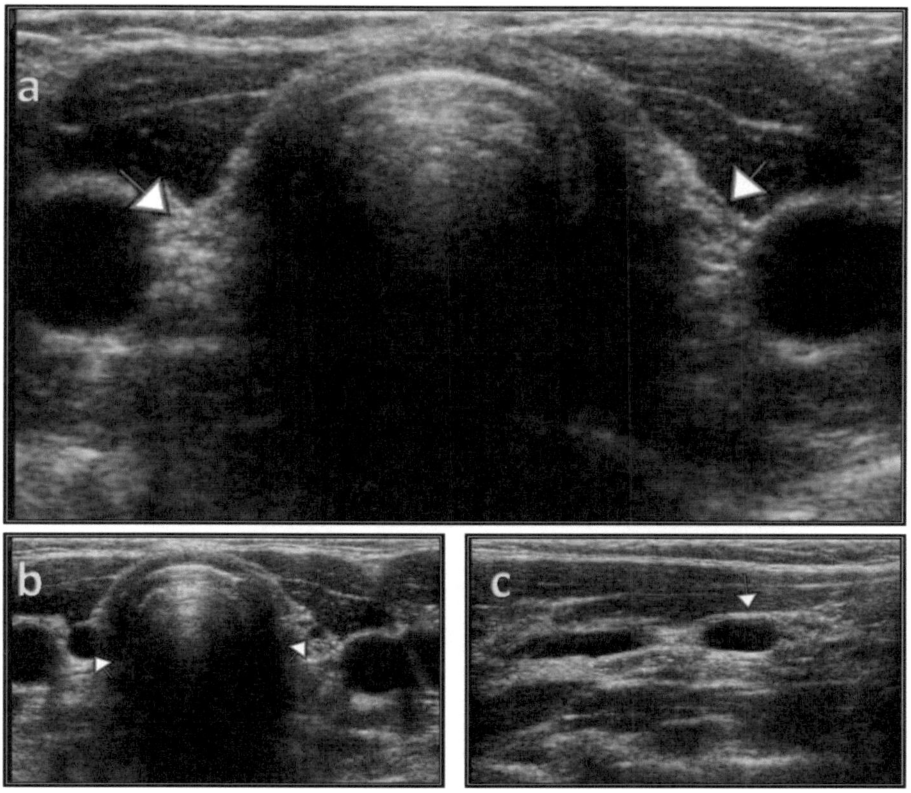

Figure 6.
(a) Athyreosis, empty thyroid lodge caused by agenesis. The arrows indicate echogenic triangles, representing ultimobranchial and connective tissue residue. (b) In the transverse and (c) sagittal planes, as in this case, there are bilateral cysts (arrows), also called ultimobranchial cysts, in the empty thyroid lodge. There is no flow on Color Doppler Imaging (not shown). (Courtesy of Prof Dr. Suat Fitoz from his archive. Department of Pediatric Radiology, Ankara University School of Medicine, Ankara/Turkey).

Due to the nature of thyroid gland embryology, when athyreoisis is detected in a patient, neck scans are required to search for the thyroid gland from the base of the tongue to the superior mediastinum in the midline on the embryological migration trace of the thyroid gland. The ectopic thyroid gland can be located in lingual, sublingual, hyoid, infrahyoid, and mediastinal. The lingual thyroid, the most common form of thyroid dysgenesis, accounts for 75% of the functioning tissues in cases of congenital hypothyroidism. On ultrasonography, ectopic thyroid tissue is well-defined oval shaped, and on color Doppler imaging it is usually hypervascular. Ectopia may initially be overlooked due to adequate hormone production in the neonatal period. In early childhood, hypothyroidism may become evident due to the increased need for thyroid hormone. Detection of the ectopic thyroid gland in scintigraphy depends on the size of the gland and whether it functions or not. Retrosternal, endolaryngeal, or endotracheal ectopic thyroids in the mediastinum are usually not detectable sonographically, in which case scintigraphic studies are required [11, 19–21]. Lingual ectopic thyroid cases are presented in **Figure** 7.

Athyreosis and residual echogenic tissues in the thyroid gland site observed in agenesis are unilateral in hemiagenesis. It can be detected incidentally in asymptomatic euthyroid patients, and in children with thyroid hemiagenesis, thyroid hormones may decrease during adolescence when the need for thyroid hormone is high. The absence of unilateral lobe and normal or goiter lobe on the opposite side can be observed on ultrasound. Scintigraphy can be used as a complement to exclude any additional orthotopic/ectopic functional thyroid tissue [20].

Thyroid hypoplasia, which is difficult to diagnose among thyroid dysgenesis, is responsible for 5% of congenital hypothyroidism cases. On ultrasound, the gland is usually hypoechoic, orthotopic (where it should be, not ectopic), normally shaped and normal in size or small for its age. Hypoplasia can be diagnosed in newborns with a tracheal index of less than 1.7 and a low uptake on scintigraphy [11]. The thyroid hemiaganesis and hypoplasia are demonstrated in **Figure 8**.

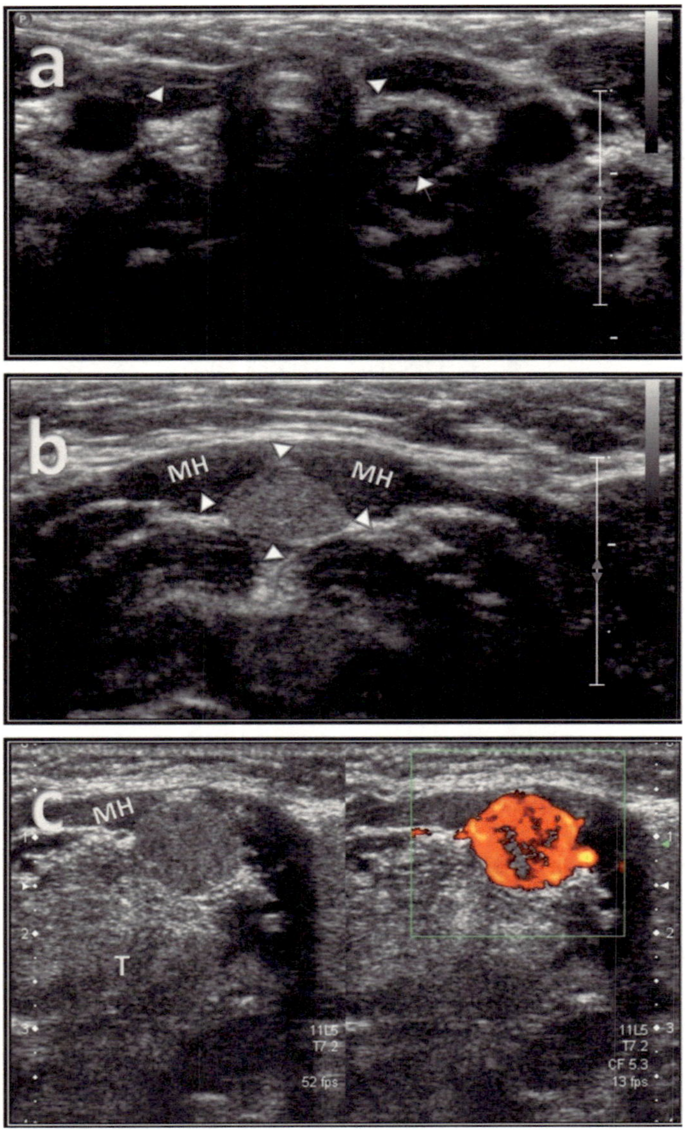

Figure 7.
(a) Athyreosis, empty thyroid lodge. The arrowsheads indicate echogenic triangles, representing ultimobranchial and connective tissue residue. The esophagus is more prominent (arrow). (b) The floor of the mouth superficial ultrasound examination, the lingual ectopic thyroid is seen as similar as normal thyroid echogenicity. (c) Another case of lingual ectopic thyroid is seen as ovoid, isoechoic, and hypervascular. (MH: Mylohyoid muscle, T: Tongue) (Courtesy of Prof Dr. Suat Fitoz from his archive. Department of Pediatric Radiology, Ankara University School of Medicine, Ankara/Turkey).

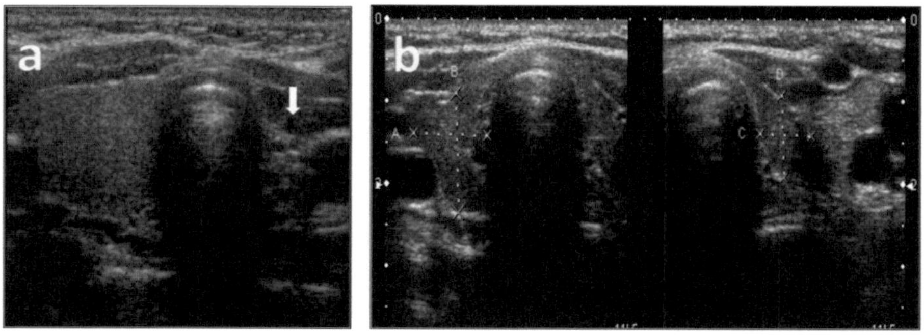

Figure 8.
(a) In hemiagenesis, athyreosis and residual echogenic tissue (arrow) is observed in the left thyroid gland site unilaterally. (b) The case of thyroid hypoplasia. The right and left lobes dimensions in the transverse plane are 11.3 and 7.9 mm, respectively. The transverse diameter of the trachea is 13,7 mm. The tracheal index was calculated as 1,4 and interpreted as hypoplasia. (Courtesy of Prof Dr. Suat Fitoz from his archive. Department of Pediatric Radiology, Ankara University School of Medicine, Ankara/Turkey).

4.2.2.2 Dyshormonogenesis

It constitutes 20% of congenital hypothyroidism. Dyshormonogenesis, in which the thyroid gland mostly has normal aspects and non-function, is characterized by defects in enzymatic processes in hormone production steps. The thyroid gland is orthotopically located. It may be of normal size and shape, or goiter may develop under thyroid-stimulating hormone. Since scintigraphic uptake may show differences due to deficiencies in different steps in dyshormonogenesis, uptake may be observed in some forms but not in some cases [20–22].

4.3 Iodine deficiency

Dietary iodine deficiency is still the most common cause of goiter and hypothyroidism in endemic areas of the world. Low hormone production after low iodine intake induces the elevation of thyroid-stimulating hormone. This causes diffuse and subsequently nodular goiter at the expense of maintaining the euthyroid state. Although iodine deficiency does not have a pathognomonic ultrasound finding, goiter with diffusely increased or multiple nodules could be detected on ultrasound.

4.4 Thyroiditis

Diffuse enlargement of the thyroid gland is a common finding. While iodine deficiency is still the most common cause of goiter and hypothyroidism worldwide, in the United States and other countries where dietary iodine intake is adequate, chronic lymphocytic thyroiditis (CLT) is the most common cause of goiter and hypothyroidism. CTL is also called Hashimoto's thyroiditis. Thyroiditis is the general definition of thyroid inflammation that can occur for many reasons. Although the spectrum of thyroiditis often overlaps in clinical, imaging, and laboratory findings, ultrasound is a very useful tool in evaluating thyroiditis as it provides information about the etiology and clinical course.

4.4.1 Chronic lymphocytic (Hashimoto's) thyroiditis (CLT)

Chronic lymphocytic thyroiditis is the most common form of thyroiditis in which autoimmunity plays a role in the pathogenesis. About 10% of the U.S. population and an estimated 25% of women over 65 exhibit antibodies to thyroid peroxidase. In Hashimoto thyroiditis, the thyroid cells are ruined through the cell and antibody-mediated immune process. The damage starts via the formation of antithyroid antibodies that attack the thyroid tissue and finally result in progressive fibrosis. Until late in the disease process, the condition is sometimes not diagnosed. The most common laboratory findings show elevated thyroid-stimulating hormone (TSH) and low thyroxine (T4) levels, along with increased antithyroid peroxidase (anti-TPO) antibodies. Women are affected 10 times more than men. The disease is frequently diagnosed between the 3rd and 5th decades [23]. The most important feature of the disease is the invasion of the thyroid gland parenchyma by lymphoplasmacytic cells. This situation reveals enlargement of the thyroid gland, heterogeneity, and diffuse decrease in echogenicity, among the most important findings on ultrasound. Sonographically, the clinical course ranges from heterogeneous and hypoechoic parenchyma to fibrosis and gland atrophy. Patients with chronic lymphocytic thyroiditis may develop primary thyroid lymphoma, representing less than 5% of all thyroid malignancies. Primary thyroid lymphoma should be suspected if an atrophic gland enlarges rapidly or especially in the presence of systemic symptoms [24].

There are studies in which high positive and negative predictive values of hypoechogenicity, indicating autoimmune disease and the risk of clinically significant hypothyroidism. It even may have an equal predictive value as the presence of thyroid autoantibodies for the development of hypothyroidism [25–28]. While positive antithyroid peroxidase antibodies are predictive of the clinical syndrome, a small subset of no more than 10–15% of the population has individuals with the clinically evident disease who are serum antibody negative [23]. Recognition of the ultrasonographic pattern of chronic lymphocytic thyroiditis in this subgroup may facilitate in determining the etiology and patient management.

4.4.1.1 Ultrasonographic patterns of Hashimoto's disease

The different appearance patterns can describe changes in CLT at different stages of the disease from early to late. The findings of chronic lymphocytic thyroiditis are presented in **Figure 9**. These patterns can be listed as hypoechoic and heterogeneous, pseudomicronodular, pseudomacronodular, markedly hypoechoic, and fibrosis-atrophy. These patterns do not represent an absolute sequential progression. Although fibrosis and atrophy are typically late manifestations, any other patterns may be seen early in the disease.

Normal thyroid tissue, as mentioned above, is hyperechoic compared to muscle tissue due to its iodine content. The thyroid gland has a uniformly homogeneous echogenicity. When the thyroid gland is exposed to lymphocytic infiltration, iodine-containing colloidal contents and normal cells in the parenchyma are destroyed. Lymphocyte infiltrates appear hypoechoic, similar to the low echo observed due to lymphocytes in lymphoid tissues. Hypoechogenicity formed by infiltrates together with normal hyperechoic areas causes a heterogeneous appearance in the gland. Both the degree of hypoechogenicity and heterogeneity varies with the distribution and severity of the lymphocytic infiltration.

When areas of hypoechoic lymphocytic infiltrate are more discrete, localized hypoechoic foci representing lymphocyte clusters are defined as pseudomicronodules. These pseudonodules are flame-shaped, hypoechogenic foci not exceeding 1 cm in size with a thin hyperechogenic fibrotic rim.

Pseudomacronodules, when the hypoechoic infiltrate areas are larger, the pseudonodules also appear larger, can often cause problems in distinguishing them from true nodules. When they are unilateral, nodule features should be examined in terms of malignancy association.

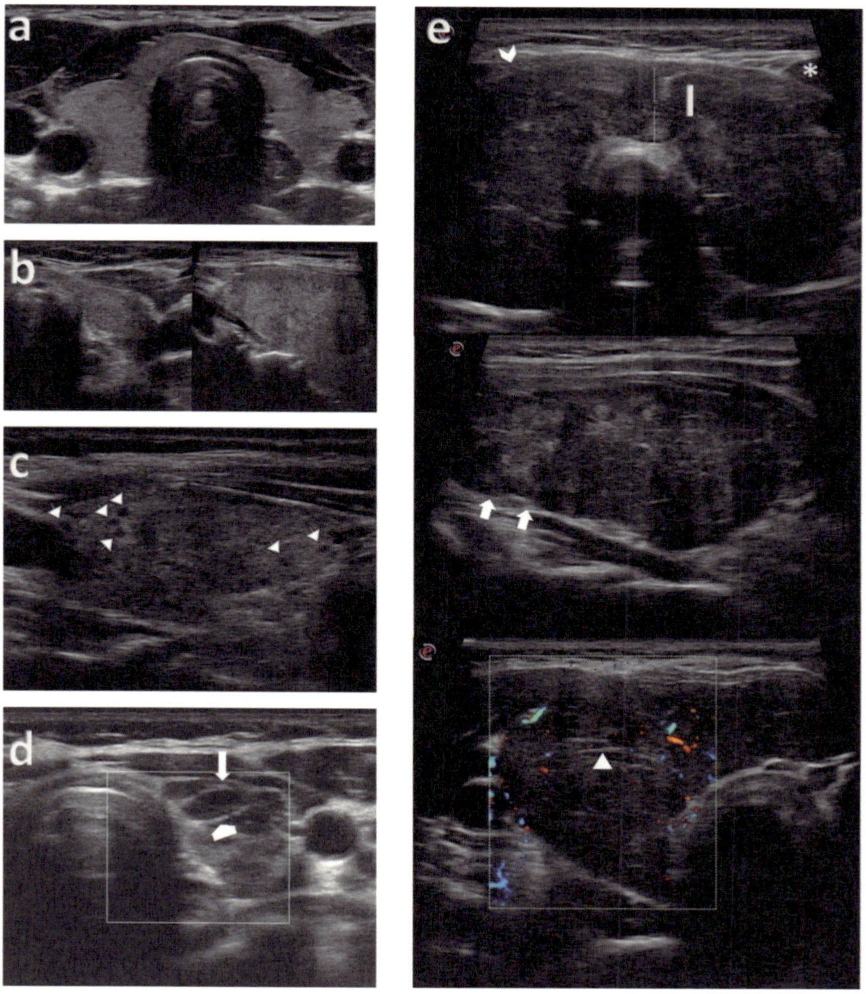

Figure 9.
Ultrasound findings of chronic lymphocytic thyroiditis. (a) The normal appearance of the gland for comparison. (b) Hypoechogenicity-heterogeneity pattern. The left lobe in the transverse and the right in the sagittal plane are shown. Hypoechogenicity formed by infiltrates and normal hyperechoic areas causes a heterogeneous appearance (relative according to a) in the gland. (c) Pseudomicronodular pattern. Hypoechoic lymphocytic infiltrate is discrete, localized hypoechoic foci (arrows) representing lymphocyte clusters are defined as pseudomicronodules that are flame-shaped, hypoechogenic foci not exceeding 1 cm in size with a thin hyperechogenic fibrotic rim. (d) Pseudomacronodular pattern. When the hypoechoic infiltrate areas are larger, the pseudonodules (arrow) also appear larger. Hyperechoic thin fibrotic septa (arrowhead) are observed in the periphery. (e) Markedly hypoechoic and fibrotic pattern. Gland sizes have increased, as can be seen from the isthmus (I) thickness. Bowing is observed in the anterior (arrowhead) of both lobes of the gland. The echogenicity of the gland is as low as the strap muscles indicated by asterisks. In the sagittal image, it is observed that the gland contours (arrows) are lobulated. In the Color Doppler Imaging, it was observed that the blood supply of the gland decreased. The thin echogenic linear formation indicated by the triangle represents fibrosis.

The markedly hypoechogenic pattern is typically seen as a large inflamed goiter. The thyroid parenchyma may be completely infiltrated with lymphocytes rather than discrete lymphocyte centres. The thyroid is equal to or more hypoechoic than adjacent muscle tissue. Thyroid lymphoma may have a very similar appearance and should be considered in the differential diagnosis, especially if there is rapid growth [24].

Finally, in the fibrosis-atrophy stage of progression of thyroid inflammation, fibrosis develops and appears sonographically as hyperechoic linear and curvilinear bands.

4.4.1.2 Doppler imaging findings of Hashimoto's disease

Color Doppler imaging (CDI) is a technique that complements the greyscale evaluation in thyroid ultrasonography and provides information about vascularity. The frequency shift that is constituted by increasing the frequency with the objects approaching the transducer and decreasing the frequency with the diverging ones, which is obtained by echoing the sound waves sent to the tissue, gives information about direction and speed. This phenomenon is also known as the "Doppler effect". CDI depends on the angle between the transducer and vessel and flow direction, whereas the "Power Doppler imaging (PDI)" is not. PDI is motion-sensitive and often amplifies the Doppler signal. It is independent of velocity, angle and flow direction. Allows slower flows to be detected with higher sensitivity than color Doppler. In the normal thyroid gland parenchyma, less than 5 vascular coding is expected in the sampling window at the lowest pulse repetition frequency (PRF) values without background noise on color Doppler ultrasound (CDI).

CDI findings may vary according to the stage of the disease. In the early and acute phase of the disease (usually in thyrotoxicosis, also known as Hashitoxicosis due to thyroid gland destruction), increased glandular blood supply may be observed, which may be due to trophic stimulation of TSH associated with the development of hypothyroidism. Doppler examination findings may show a diffuse hypervascularization pattern similar to Graves' disease during this time period. A decrease in Doppler signals will be observed in the advanced stages due to intense fibrosis and avascularity in Doppler examination. The Hashitoxicosis case is shown in **Figure 10**.

In Hashimoto's disease, there are cases with negative autoantibodies and hypothyroidism and a group with positive autoantibodies but without overt hypothyroidism. Sonographic and Doppler findings similar to Hashimoto's disease can be observed in euthyroid patients with positive anti-TPO autoantibodies. A study by Acar et al. found that only euthyroid individuals with high levels of antithyroid autoantibodies had similar sonographic structural and hemodynamic characteristics on Doppler examination, as observed in patients with Hashimoto's disease with hypothyroidism. They thought that structural and hemodynamic changes could begin much earlier than symptoms and hormonal imbalance [29].

4.4.1.3 Lymph nodes and microcalcifications in Hashimoto's disease

In the presence of Hashimoto's thyroiditis, one of the most common conditions encountered in thyroid ultrasonography is lymph nodes found in the central lymph node compartment and at levels III and IV. Knowing the characteristics of disease-associated reactive enlarging lymph nodes is important to avoid invasive unnecessary biopsies to rule out metastatic or lymphoproliferative diseases. A healthy lymph node consists of a hilum with fatty content and afferent-efferent vessels, which is hyperechoic on ultrasonography, and a more hypoechoic cortex with a thickness of less than 3 mm. Normal shape is fusiform. The normal ranges of lymph node sizes vary according to the station where the lymph node is located, and cut-off values are highly controversial. They are defined by the long and short axis dimensions obtained perpendicular to each other in the plane where the lymph node appears longest. Although there is no clear rule, 1 cm above the short axis is diagnosed pathologically in head and neck ultrasonography. As the short axis cut-off values get smaller, the sensitivity increases, and the specificity decreases, causing extra and unnecessary invasive procedures. Rather than the length of the short axis, the shape of the lymph node, the thickness of the cortex, and whether the fatty hilum can be distinguished are more important in defining the pathologies.

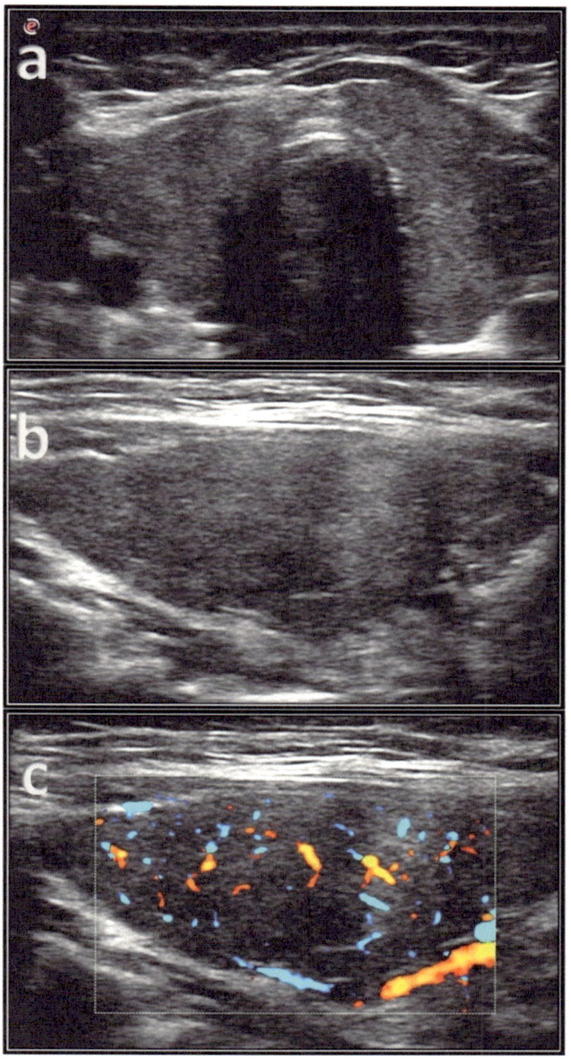

Figure 10.
A 37-year-old female patient is admitted with low TSH and high T4. In the thyroid ultrasound performed, (a) Diffuse decrease in echogenicity of the thyroid gland is observed in the transverse plane, and its echotexture is heterogeneous. (b) Similar findings are observed in the sagittal image. (c) Here, an increase in vascularity is observed in Color Doppler Imaging, which may be in the early or acute phase of the disease. The patient was diagnosed with Hashitoxicosis with clinical-laboratory and ultrasonographic findings.

Whether it is a metastatic or lymphoproliferative disease, infection or inflammatory processes such as Hashimoto, the lymph nodes become larger and more prominent. However, pathology is highly recognizable due to nuance differences such as shape, echo pattern and existence of fatty hilus. These features increase success in choosing the right patient for further examination.

It is lymph node enlargement, defined as reactive lymph node enlargement, defined in infectious and inflammatory diseases such as Hashimoto's. In fact, this is a diagnosis of exclusion. This name is given to lymph node enlargements in which malignant features such as ovoid or round shape, the fatty hilum could not be distinguished as hyperechoic due to infiltration, and blood supply from outside the hilum are excluded. The reactive lymph node should be fusiform, have a homogeneous hypoechoic cortex, and the fatty hilus should be distinguishable

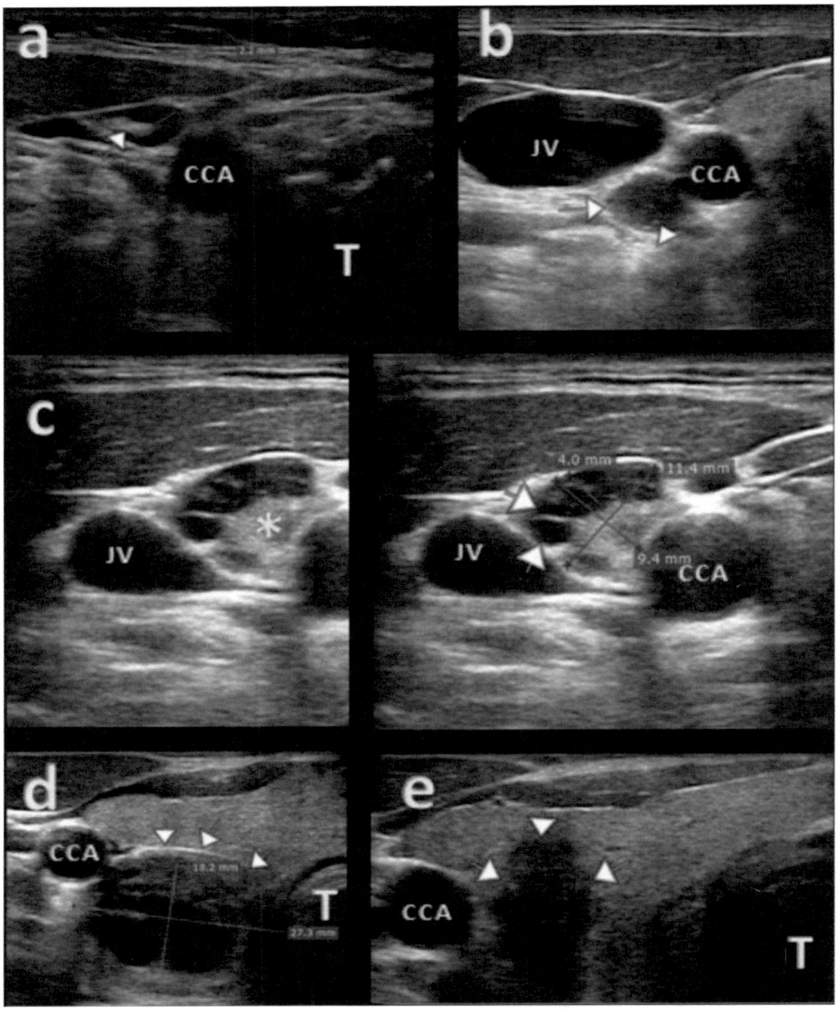

Figure 11.
Examples of lymph nodes that may be encountered during thyroid ultrasonography examination. a) Enlarged reactive lymph node at right cervical level III (most commonly observed in the pretracheal area, not shown here) secondary to the inflammatory process in Hashimoto's disease. Distinguishable hyperechoic fatty hilus marked with arrow. Homogeneous, hypoechoic cortex thinner than 3 mm. b-e) Images aquised from another patient. b) A pathologically enlarged lymph node (arrow) in the right cervical level III-IV, with a round shaped, hyperechogenic fatty hilus indistinguishable, with a small echogenic focus compatible with microcalcification (arrowhead). c) At right cervical level III, although the short axis is shorter than 1 cm (9.4 mm) and the fatty hilus (asteriks) can be distinguished, pathological lymph node is characterized by a heterogeneous and thicker (4 mm) than 3 mm cortex with cystic areas (arrows). d) Further inferiorly, at the right cervical level IV. Pathologically enlarged lymph node with cystic-solid component, with a short axis (18.2 mm) greater than 1 cm, preserved fat plane (arrows) intermediate with the thyroid, e) The source of all these metastatic lymph nodes is a malignant thyroid nodule located in the right lobe, with lobulated contour, markedly hypoechoic compared to the strap muscle, and taller-than-wide shaped. FNA was performed and the diagnosis of papillary thyroid cancer was confirmed cytopathologically.

as hyperechoic. Microcalcification and cystic changes (unless abscess formation secondary to suppurative lymphadenitis) is not observed in reactive lymph node enlargement. In this case, the pathognomonic findings of papillary thyroid cancer metastasis are considered, and it is necessary to look for a malignant nodule in the thyroid. In addition, reactive lymph nodes enlargements in Hashimoto's disease are located in the pretracheal and perithyroidal areas. In **Figure 11**, lymph nodes detected in thyroid ultrasonography examinations are observed.

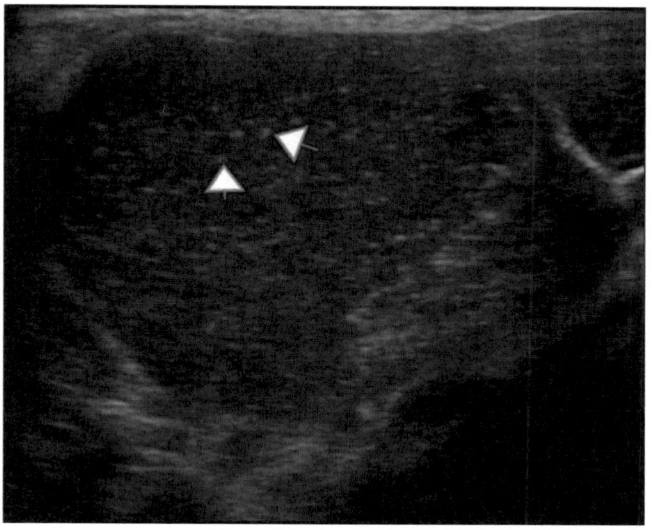

Figure 12.
Thyroid ultrasonography of a patient with Hashimoto's disease. At right lobe, numerous hyperechoic foci with a markedly hypoechoic background, 1–2 mm in size, with no acoustic shadow consistent with microcalcification (arrows). Biopsy was performed to rule out malignancy. The pathology result was reported as chronic lymphocytic thyroiditis.

One of the uncommon manifestations of Hashimoto's disease is diffuse microcalcifications. Microcalcifications are recognized as hyperechogenic foci with a 1–2 mm diameter that do not produce a posterior acoustic shadow. Undoubtedly, one of the pathognomonic findings of papillary thyroid cancer is microcalcification. Since it is a cancer finding, it causes diagnostic difficulties with its detection in Hashimoto's disease and makes fine needle biopsy mandatory to exclude malignancy. Especially when it is difficult to distinguish the pseudonodule from the true nodule, it may cause greater confusion. Cytopathological findings guide the correct diagnosis in such cases. The microcalcification in Hashimoto's Disease is shown in **Figure 12**.

4.4.2 Subacute granulomatous (De Quervain) thyroiditis

DeQuervain or subacute thyroiditis occurs due to the immune response following a viral or upper respiratory tract infection. The disease is often self-limited. However, its clinical presentation is an acute painful neck with systemic symptoms such as tender goiter, fever, fatigue, weight loss, high erythrocyte sedimentation rate or C-reactive protein, suppressed TSH level, and dysphagia. Patients may be hyperthyroid in the acute phase but usually become hypothyroid until they return to the euthyroid state after about 6 to 18 months. The typical ultrasound appearance of the gland is characterized by decreased vascularity of patchy, ill-defined hypoechoic areas in one or both lobes with involvement of the thyroid parenchyma. Sometimes the appearance is described as "lava flow" with diffuse and combined hypoechoic areas. Thus, the acute phase may show hypervascularity, while the subacute phase may reflect diffuse hypovascularity. The case of subacute granulomatous thyroiditis is demonstrated in **Figure 13**.

4.4.3 Painless thyroiditis (silent thyroiditis-postpartum thyroiditis)

Painless thyroiditis is a symptom-based classification, which includes both silent thyroiditis and postpartum thyroiditis. Silent thyroiditis is autoimmune and

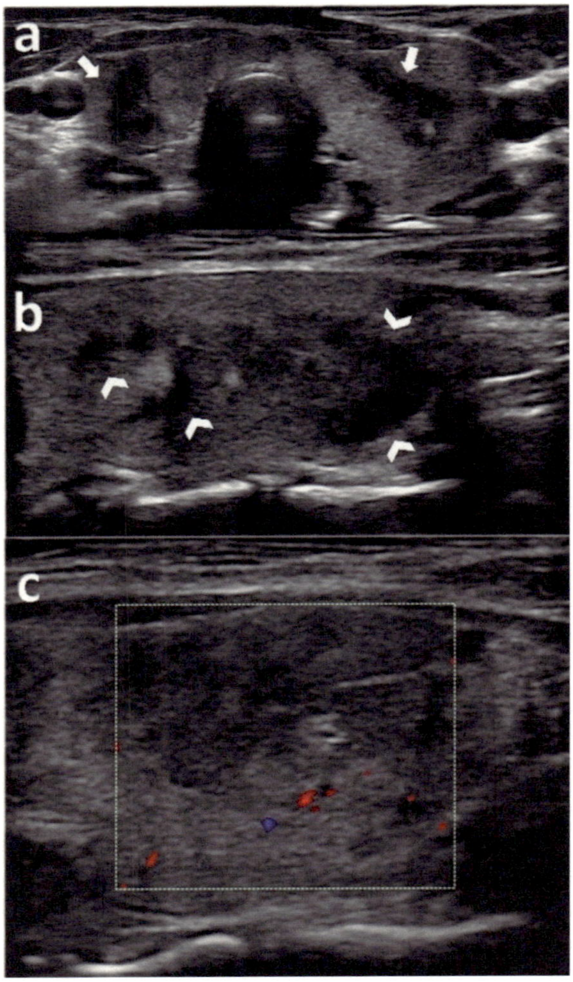

Figure 13.
A 40-year-old female patient presented with pain and tenderness in the anterior neck and general fatigue. It is understood from her history that he had a viral upper respiratory tract infection 2 weeks ago. Laboratory findings were high erythrocyte sedimentation rate, C-reactive protein and low TSH level. In the ultrasound; (a) In the transverse plane, there is an appearance like a focal nodular hypoechoic lesion (arrows) with unclear borders in both lobes. (b) The sagittal view of the left lobe shows that the lesion extends and spreads craniocaudal. Thus, with this finding, it was first understood that this was not a true nodule. Thyroiditis was considered as a preliminary diagnosis. Patchy hypoechoic areas are likened to "lava flows". (c) In addition, decreased blood supply in thyroiditis areas, as observed in Color Doppler examination, is another finding helpful in the diagnosis. It was diagnosed as De Quervain thyroiditis with clinical-laboratory and ultrasonographic findings.

considered a temporary form of Hashimoto's thyroiditis. They have lower thyroid autoantibody levels than those seen in Hashimoto's thyroiditis and frequently seen in women aged 30–50 years. Postpartum thyroiditis got this name because it occurs within 1 year after birth. It is seen in 10% of all pregnancies, and the recurrence rate in subsequent pregnancies is up to 70%. Patients may present either in the thyrotoxic phase, which is usually mild and lasts for 1–2 months or in the hypothyroid phase, typically transient, lasting 4–6 months. On ultrasound, hypoechogenicity is observed, as in other forms of autoimmune thyroid disease. Unlike Hashimoto's, hyperechoic fibrotic bands and marked hypoechogenicity are usually absent [30].

4.4.4 Suppurative thyroiditis

This type is a rare infection caused by a bacterial pathogen, seen in immunocompromised patients or children and young adults with branchial anomalies. A euthyroid patient may present with inflammation such as fever, sore throat, painful swelling, skin erythema, and lymphadenopathy. On ultrasound, an increase in blood supply to the thyroid gland is usually observed. Sometimes abscess formation can be observed [30].

5. Follow-up

The necessity of the ultrasonographic follow-up of the thyroid gland for hypothyroidism is debatable. However, when the antibodies are negative in the suspected cases, the ultrasonographic process of thyroiditis may be the sole evidence for chronic lymphocytic thyroiditis. Pattern recognition is a tool for diagnosis in such cases. In addition, subclinical hypothyroidism that may need treatment and other non-chronic thyroiditis outcomes can be determined by ultrasonographic follow-up.

Another follow-up reason is for malignancy that is occurred as papillary thyroid cancer (PTC) and primary thyroid lymphoma. Publications are showing that both malignancies are associated with hypothyroidism. Along with hypothyroidism, PTC suspected nodules have the same features (hypoechogenicity, microcalcifications, taller than wide shape etc) regardless of thyroid hormone state. The key role of the follow-up in hypothyroidism is that the nodule is true whether or not. If a new nodule develops malignance should be ruled out. Thereby the recording and the comparison with the old image is precious. Another malignancy is primary thyroid lymphoma. The risk increases with chronic lymphocytic thyroiditis. Once lymphocytes diffusely infiltrate the thyroid gland, the thyroid is equal to or more hypoechoic than adjacent muscle tissue. Thyroid lymphoma may have a very similar appearance and should be considered in the differential diagnosis, especially if there is rapid growth. It is often not easy to distinguish between the two situations. Therefore, the correlation of sonographic findings with systemic symptoms is important.

6. Conclusion

Ultrasonography is an indispensable complementary tool in hypothyroidism, which can be seen in almost all ages, from fetal life to geriatric age groups. Knowing the characteristic ultrasonographic findings of Hashimoto's disease, which is the most common cause of hypothyroidism in areas without iodine deficiency, is very important in diagnosis, especially in patients with negative thyroid autoantibodies. Hypoechogenicity should be remembered that it is the key finding in hypothyroidism. Such that; the predictive value is equal to that of autoantibodies. Another point that should not be overlooked when evaluating the thyroid gland is the cervical lymph nodes. Lymph nodes may reactively enlarge in diseases such as Hashimoto's disease as in malignancies. Rather than the size of the lymph node in the differentiation of reactive-malignancy, findings favoring reactive lymph node enlargements, such as fusiform shape, distinguishable echogenic fatty hilum, blood supply only from the hilum, homogeneous and thin cortex, and no changes such as cystic or microcalcification. Otherwise, a biopsy should be performed to exclude malignancy. One of the uncommon manifestations of Hashimoto's disease is diffuse microcalcifications. It causes diagnostic difficulties with its detection in Hashimoto's disease and makes fine needle biopsy mandatory to exclude malignancy. Although the details of the thyroid gland can be demonstrated by ultrasonography alone, it can never replace the evaluation of ultrasonography reinforced with clinical knowledge. This synergy will be possible by increasing interdisciplinary communication.

Author details

Hakan Baş
Department of Radiology, Occupational and Environmental Diseases Hospital, Ankara, Turkey

*Address all correspondence to: hakanbas7@outlook.com

References

[1] Patil N, Rehman A, Jialal I. Hypothyroidism. StatPearls. Treasure Island (FL): StatPearls Publishing Copyright © 2021, StatPearls Publishing LLC.; 2021.

[2] Fujimoto Y, Oka A, Omoto R, Hirose M. Ultrasound scanning of the thyroid gland as a new diagnostic approach. Ultrasonics. 1967;5(3):177-180.

[3] Milas M, Mandel SJ, Langer JE. Advanced Thyroid and Parathyroid Ultrasound. 2017.

[4] The thyroid nodule. Ann Intern Med. 1982;96(2):221-32.

[5] AIUM-ACR-SPR-SRU Practice Parameter for the Performance and Interpretation of a Diagnostic Ultrasound Examination of the Extracranial Head and Neck. J Ultrasound Med. 2018;37(11):E6-E12.

[6] Richman DM, Frates MC. Ultrasound of the Normal Thyroid with Technical Pearls and Pitfalls. Radiol Clin North Am. 2020;58(6):1033-1039.

[7] Blum M. Ultrasonography of the Thyroid. In: Feingold KR, Anawalt B, Boyce A, Chrousos G, de Herder WW, Dhatariya K, et al., editors. Endotext. South Dartmouth (MA): MDText.com, Inc.Copyright © 2000-2021, MDText.com, Inc.; 2000.

[8] Chanoine JP, Toppet V, Lagasse R, Spehl M, Delange F. Determination of thyroid volume by ultrasound from the neonatal period to late adolescence. Eur J Pediatr. 1991;150(6):395-399.

[9] Zimmermann MB, Hess SY, Molinari L, De Benoist B, Delange F, Braverman LE, et al. New reference values for thyroid volume by ultrasound in iodine-sufficient schoolchildren: a World Health Organization/Nutrition for Health and Development Iodine Deficiency Study Group Report. Am J Clin Nutr. 2004;79(2):231-237.

[10] Moradi M, Hashemipour M, Akbari S, Kor Z, Mirbod SA, Kooshanmehr MR. Ultrasonographic evaluation of the thyroid gland volume among 8-15-year-old children in Isfahan, Iran. Adv Biomed Res. 2014;3:9.

[11] Goldis M, Waldman L, Marginean O, Rosenberg HK, Rapaport R. Thyroid Imaging in Infants. Endocrinol Metab Clin North Am. 2016;45(2):255-266.

[12] Yasumoto M, Inoue H, Ohashi I, Shibuya H, Onishi T. Simple new technique for sonographic measurement of the thyroid in neonates and small children. J Clin Ultrasound. 2004;32(2):82-85.

[13] Hollowell JG, Staehling NW, Flanders WD, Hannon WH, Gunter EW, Spencer CA, et al. Serum TSH, T(4), and thyroid antibodies in the United States population (1988 to 1994): National Health and Nutrition Examination Survey (NHANES III). J Clin Endocrinol Metab. 2002;87(2): 489-499.

[14] Ranzini AC, Ananth CV, Smulian JC, Kung M, Limbachia A, Vintzileos AM. Ultrasonography of the fetal thyroid: nomograms based on biparietal diameter and gestational age. J Ultrasound Med. 2001;20(6):613-617.

[15] Agrawal P, Ogilvy-Stuart A, Lees C. Intrauterine diagnosis and management of congenital goitrous hypothyroidism. Ultrasound Obstet Gynecol. 2002;19(5):501-505.

[16] Khater C, Ceccaldi PF, Poujade O, Banigé M, Ottenwalter A, Luton D. Foetal thyroid dysfunction: treat the mother first! Horm Res Paediatr. 2015;83(2):136-140.

[17] Silva CT, Navarro OM. Pearls and Pitfalls in Pediatric Thyroid Imaging. Seminars in Ultrasound, CT and MRI. 2020;41(5):421-432.

[18] Sedassari AdA, de Souza LRMF, Sedassari NdA, Borges MdF, Palhares HMdC, de Andrade Neto GB. Sonographic evaluation of children with congenital hypothyroidism. Radiol Bras. 2015;48(4):220-224.

[19] Karakoc-Aydiner E, Turan S, Akpinar I, Dede F, Isguven P, Adal E, et al. Pitfalls in the diagnosis of thyroid dysgenesis by thyroid ultrasonography and scintigraphy. European Journal of Endocrinology. 2012;166(1):43-48.

[20] Hong HS, Lee EH, Jeong SH, Park J, Lee H. Ultrasonography of various thyroid diseases in children and adolescents: a pictorial essay. Korean J Radiol. 2015;16(2):419-429.

[21] Chang YW, Hong HS, Choi DL. Sonography of the pediatric thyroid: a pictorial essay. J Clin Ultrasound. 2009;37(3):149-157.

[22] Williams JL, Paul DL, Bisset G, 3rd. Thyroid disease in children: part 1: State-of-the-art imaging in pediatric hypothyroidism. Pediatr Radiol. 2013;43(10):1244-1253.

[23] Mincer DL, Jialal I. Hashimoto Thyroiditis. StatPearls. Treasure Island (FL): StatPearls Publishing Copyright © 2021, StatPearls Publishing LLC.; 2021.

[24] Kesireddy M, Lasrado S. Thyroid Lymphoma.

[25] Pedersen OM, Aardal NP, Larssen TB, Varhaug JE, Myking O, Vik-Mo H. The value of ultrasonography in predicting autoimmune thyroid disease. Thyroid. 2000;10(3):251-259.

[26] Raber W, Gessl A, Nowotny P, Vierhapper H. Thyroid ultrasound versus antithyroid peroxidase antibody determination: a cohort study of four hundred fifty-one subjects. Thyroid. 2002;12(8):725-731.

[27] Rago T, Chiovato L, Grasso L, Pinchera A, Vitti P. Thyroid ultrasonography as a tool for detecting thyroid autoimmune diseases and predicting thyroid dsfunction in apparently healthy subjects. J Endocrinol Invest. 2001;24(10):763-769.

[28] Rotondi M, Cappelli C, Leporati P, Chytiris S, Zerbini F, Fonte R, et al. A hypoechoic pattern of the thyroid at ultrasound does not indicate autoimmune thyroid diseases in patients with morbid obesity. Eur J Endocrinol. 2010;163(1):105-109.

[29] Acar T, Ozbek SS, Erdogan M, Ozgen AG, Demirel SO. US findings in euthyroid patients with positive antithyroid autoantibody tests compared to normal and hypothyroid cases. Diagn Interv Radiol. 2013;19(4):265-270.

[30] Dighe M, Barr R, Bojunga J, Cantisani V, Chammas MC, Cosgrove D, et al. Thyroid Ultrasound: State of the Art Part 1 - Thyroid Ultrasound reporting and Diffuse Thyroid Diseases. Med Ultrason. 2017;19(1):79-93.

Chapter 5

Melatonin Modulates Hypophyseal-Thyroid Function through Differential Activation of MT1 and MT2 Receptors in Hypothyroid Mice

Shiv Shankar Singh, Prashanjit Laskar, Anindita Deb and Sangita Sutradhar

Abstract

Hypothyroidism is characterized by the low level of thyroid hormones in circulation, which affects the normal metabolic activities of organisms. Propylthiouracil (PTU) induced hypothyroid condition impairs the antioxidant defense system and therefore normal physiology alters. Melatonin influences most physiological activities and is also known for its antioxidative properties. Melatonin modulates physiological activities through receptor-mediated as well as non-receptor-mediated pathways. In this study, we evaluated the involvement of melatonin MT1 and MT2 receptors in the modulation of hypophyseal-thyroid function in PTU-induced hypothyroid mice. We have noted the decreased level of T3 and T4 and increased level of TSH hormone in PTU-treated mice. Melatonin treatment counteracted the PTU-caused changes in circulatory T3, T4, and TSH hormones. PTU treatment caused increased MT1 receptor protein expression in the thyroid as well as the pituitary gland while increased MT2 receptor protein in the pituitary gland. Melatonin treatment caused increased TSH receptor protein in the thyroid gland. Melatonin induced MT2 receptor protein expression in both the thyroid and pituitary glands whereas MT1 receptor proteins in the pituitary gland. This study may suggest that melatonin regulates hypophyseal-thyroid function through differential sensitization of MT1 and MT2 receptors on the pituitary and thyroid glands in hypothyroid mice.

Keywords: melatonin, propylthiouracil, pituitary, thyroid, hypothyroid, melatonin receptors

1. Introduction

Thyroid hormones play a vital role in the physiology of the organism by influencing almost all tissues to grow and it maintains normal cognition, cardiovascular function, bone health, metabolism, and energy balance. Pathological disorders in the thyroid gland bring about functional changes in different organs of the body. The cardiovascular derangements were observed after the altered action of thyroid hormone on certain molecular pathways in the heart and relevant vasculature [1, 2].

Hypothyroidism is a clinical syndrome caused by decreased thyroid activity. Hypothyroidism has been associated with a sub-metabolic state with lowered energy and oxygen metabolism [3]. PTU-induced hypothyroidism impairs the antioxidant defense system as well as the physiological system of gonads during development and maturation in Wistar rats [4]. Perinatal disruption of thyroid function leads to disorders in physiological networks, including the central nervous system [5] and the immune system [6]. Development of hypothyroidism through the ingestion of methimazole or propylthiouracil in maternal rats resulted in the transfer of these drugs to the offspring and induction of several immunological changes, including a relative increase in the proportion of Treg cells in the spleen [7].

Hypothyroidism also led to changes in oxidant and antioxidant systems [8–10]. Further, neuronal developmental pattern related to oxidative stress and the antioxidant system was also affected in rat offspring by maternal hypothyroidism [11]. Melatonin hormone has antioxidative properties and protects membrane lipids, cytoplasmic proteins, and nuclear DNA [12]. Moreover, melatonin stimulates gene expression and the activity of the antioxidant enzymes glutathione peroxidase, superoxide dismutase, and catalase [13–15]. According to Thakkar et al. [16], melatonin performs the synergistic, cumulative, or antagonistic effects through which it institutes the effects of thyroid deficiency in the neonatal period of a rat.

However, melatonin mediates most of its physiological effects including modulation of immune function through activation of G-protein coupled MT1 and MT2 cell surface receptors. Further, melatonin receptors are also localized on various tissues and cells including the thyroid follicular and parafollicular cells. But how melatonin receptors are responding to the modulation of pituitary-thyroid function in the hypothyroid condition has not been studied. Therefore, in this study, we made an attempt to explore the effect of melatonin on modulation of MT1 and MT2 receptor protein expression pattern and hypophyseal-thyroid function in experimentally induced hypothyroid mice.

2. Materials and methods

All of the experiments with animals and their maintenance have been done according to the institutional practice and with the framework of CPCSEA (Committee for the Purpose of Control and Supervision of Experimental Animals) and the Act of Government of India (2007) for the animal welfare.

2.1 Experimental design

Healthy mice colony was housed at ambient laboratories conditions (under 12L:12D cycles and 25 ± 2°C temperature). Mice were kept in groups of five in polycarbonate cages (43 cm × 27 cm × 14 cm) to avoid the population stress and were fed regularly with mice feed and water *ad libitum*. Healthy male Swiss-albino mice were selected from the housed colony and were divided into five groups having five mice in each.

Group I	Control (Con)
Group II	Melatonin (Mel)
Group III	Propylthiouracil (PTU)
Group IV	(Mel + PTU)

The control group of mice received ethanolic saline (0.01% ethanol), 0.1 mL/day for consecutive 30 days. The second group of mice received subcutaneous injections of melatonin (Sigma-Aldrich Chemicals, St. Louis, USA), 25 μg/100 g BW/day for consecutive 30 days during evening (4:30–5:00 pm) hours. The third group of mice received 5-propyl-2-thiouracil, PTU (Sigma-Aldrich Chemicals, St. Louis, USA) in the drinking water, 60 μg/g BW/day for consecutive 18 days [17]. The fourth group of mice received melatonin for consecutive 30 days and also received PTU for the last 18 days of the experimental period of melatonin treatment.

After 24 h of last administration, experimental mice were sacrificed under anesthesia (pentobarbital, 15 mg/kg, intraperitoneal injection) and trunk blood was collected. Serum was separated and stored at −20°C until analyzed. Experimental tissues (pituitary and thyroid) were dissected out on the ice. One part of the thyroid gland was fixed in Bouin's for histological analysis. Thyroid and pituitary glands were stored at −20°C for Western blot analysis.

2.2 Hormonal analysis

The levels of T3, T4, and TSH hormones in the blood were tested using commercial ELISA kits (Diagnostic Automation Inc., USA) as directed by the manufacturer. T3 has a detection range of 0–10 ng/mL, with a specificity of 96.30% and a sensitivity of 0.2 ng/mL. T4 has a detection range of 0–30 μg/dL, with a sensitivity of 0.05 g/mL and a specificity of 96.30 percent. TSH had a detection range of 0–40 IU/mL, a 100% specificity, and a sensitivity of 0.20 IU/mL.

2.3 Histology

Thyroid glands were fixed overnight in Bouin's fixative and processed for paraffin block preparation and sectioning. Mayer's albumin-coated slide was used to stretch sections of 5 μm thickness. Routine hematoxylin–eosin double staining procedures were used to stain thyroid sections. Stained sections of the thyroid gland were examined under the 40X objective of Olympus BX-41 Microscope and micrographs were taken.

2.4 Western blot analysis

Tissues were homogenized in RIPA buffer (NP-40 (1%, v/v), sodium dodecyl sulfate (SDS) (1%, v/v) in PBS supplemented with phenylmethyl sulphonyl fluoride (PMSF), sodium orthovanadate and aprotinin). The total protein content of the sample was determined using the Lowry method [18]. Protein aliquots (100 μg) were resolved on a 10% (w/v) SDS polyacrylamide gel and electrotransferred to nitrocellulose membrane (Santa Cruz Biotech, USA). Primary antibodies (sc-13186, Mel 1AR (MT1); sc-13177, Mel 1BR (MT2); sc-7818, TSH-R; goat IgG, diluted 1:200; and sc-130656, β-actin antibody, rabbit IgG, Santacruz Biotech, USA, diluted 1:500) were used for immune detection. Primary antibodies were diluted in 5% skimmed milk in PBS containing 0.01% Tween-20. Secondary antibodies (goat anti-rabbit IgG-HRP and rabbit anti-goat IgG-HRP, diluted 1:1000) were used. Super Signal West Pico Chemiluminescent Substrate (#34080, Thermo Scientific, Rockford, USA) was used to identify immunological interactions. Scion Image Analysis Software (Scion Corporation, MD, USA) was used to determine the optical density measurement of the band intensity. The ratio of the specific signal to β-actin signal density was determined and presented as the % control value [19].

2.5 Statistical analysis

Statistical analysis of the data was performed using SPSS 17.0 (SPSS Corp., USA) program with one-way ANOVA followed by Tukey's honest significant difference (HSD) multiple range test. The differences were considered significant when $p < 0.05$.

3. Results

3.1 Effect of melatonin on serum level of T_3 and T_4 hormones

In this study, 5-propylthiouracil (PTU) was used to induce hypothyroid condition in experimental mice. 5-propylthiouracil interacts with the thyroid peroxidase enzyme and inhibits its activity. Thyroid peroxidase is an important enzyme involved in the iodination of tyrosine amino acids present in thyroglobulin at the luminal surface of follicular cells. Further, random coupling of iodinated tyrosine produces triiodothyronine (T3) and tetraiodothyronine (T4) on thyroglobulin on the luminal surface of follicular cells. Treatment of PTU caused significant ($p < 0.01$) suppression of circulatory T3 and T4 levels in mice (**Figures 1** and **2**). The persistent low level of T3 and T4 caused hypothyroid pathology in mice. PTU is a known antithyroid drug and is used for the treatment of hyperthyroidism in human beings. Melatonin treatment to healthy mice caused significant ($p < 0.01$) suppression of circulatory T3 and T4 levels, whereas melatonin treatment to hypothyroid groups of mice caused a significant ($p < 0.01$) increase of both T3 and T4 hormone levels.

3.2 Effect of melatonin on anatomical changes in the thyroid gland

Thyroid gland is a bilobed structure present on the trachea at apposition below the cricoid cartilage. In mammals, both lobes of the thyroid gland are joined by a

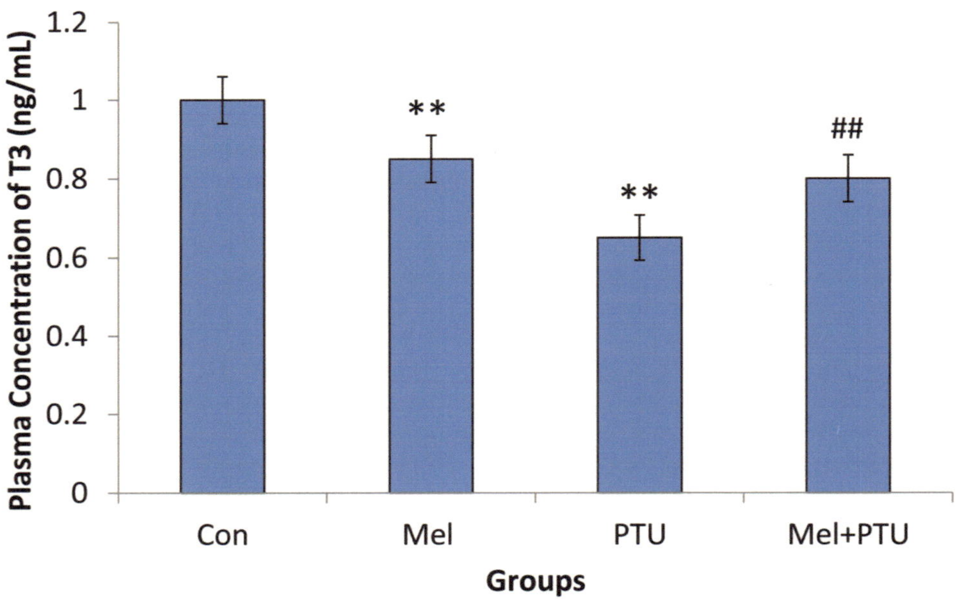

Figure 1.
Plasma T_3 concentration of experimental groups of mice. Histogram represents mean ± SEM. The mean differences were considered significant when $p < 0.01$. $^{**}p < 0.01$: Con vs. Mel; Con vs. PTU; $^{\#\#}p < 0.01$: PTU vs. Mel + PTU.

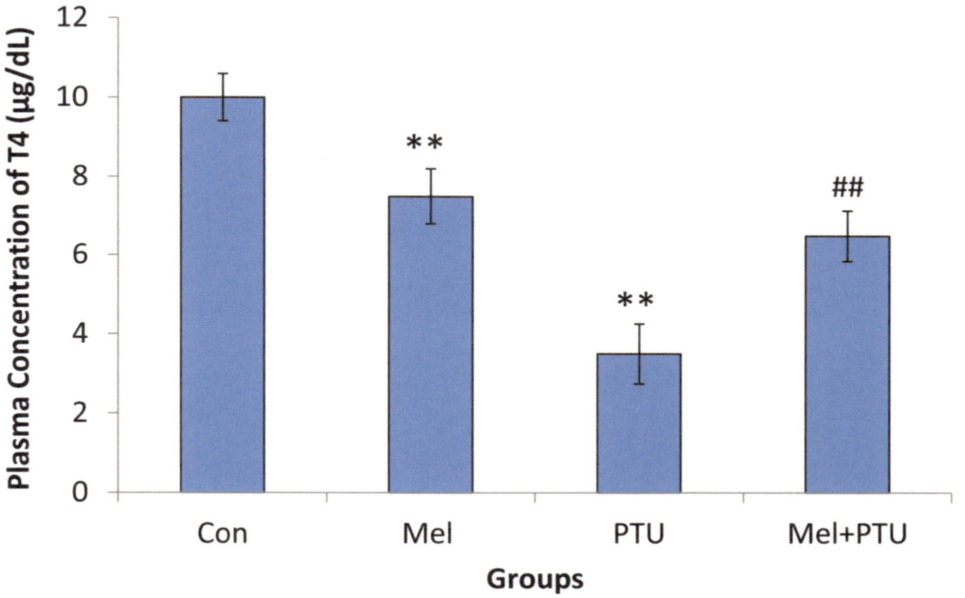

Figure 2.
Serum T_4 concentration of experimental groups of mice. Histogram represents mean ± SEM. The mean differences were considered significant when $p < 0.01$. $^{**}p < 0.01$: Con vs. Mel; Con vs. PTU; $^{\#\#}p < 0.01$: PTU vs. Mel + PTU.

narrow isthmus of tissue. Anatomically, the thyroid gland consists of follicles surrounded by a single layer of cuboidal epithelium. These thyroid follicles are a functional unit of the thyroid gland. These follicles contain lumens, which are filled with colloid materials. This colloid contains iodinated thyronine (i.e., 3,5,3′5′-tetraiodothyronine, T_4 and 3,5,3′-triiodothyronine, T_3) and iodinated tyrosine (3-monoiodotyrosine, MIT and 3,5-diiodotyrosine, DIT) on thyroglobulin molecule. In the control mice, normal size of follicles filled with colloid was observed. PTU-induced hypothyroid mice showed the abnormal shape of thyroid follicles with enlarged follicular cells (**Figure 3**). Follicles were observed with the small size of the luminal area. Melatonin-treated mice showed a normal size of thyroidal follicles. Melatonin-treated hypothyroid mice showed restoration of thyroidal follicles.

3.3 Effect of melatonin on serum TSH level and TSH receptor protein in the thyroid gland

Melatonin regulates the circadian rhythmicity of the neuroendocrine secretion. Melatonin also affects the secretory activity of the pituitary-thyroid axis. Serum TSH hormone level remains unaltered, whereas TSH receptor expression in the thyroid gland increased after melatonin treatment (**Figures 4** and **5**). PTU treatment increased the circulatory TSH hormone but TSH receptor expression in the thyroid gland remained unaffected. In melatonin-supplemented hypothyroid mice, TSH hormone level increased, whereas TSH receptor expression on the thyroid gland was unchanged in comparison with the hypothyroid group.

3.4 Effect of melatonin on MT1 and MT2 receptor proteins in the thyroid gland

Melatonin treatment significantly decreased the MT1 receptor protein in the thyroid gland whereas it significantly increased the MT2 receptor protein in the

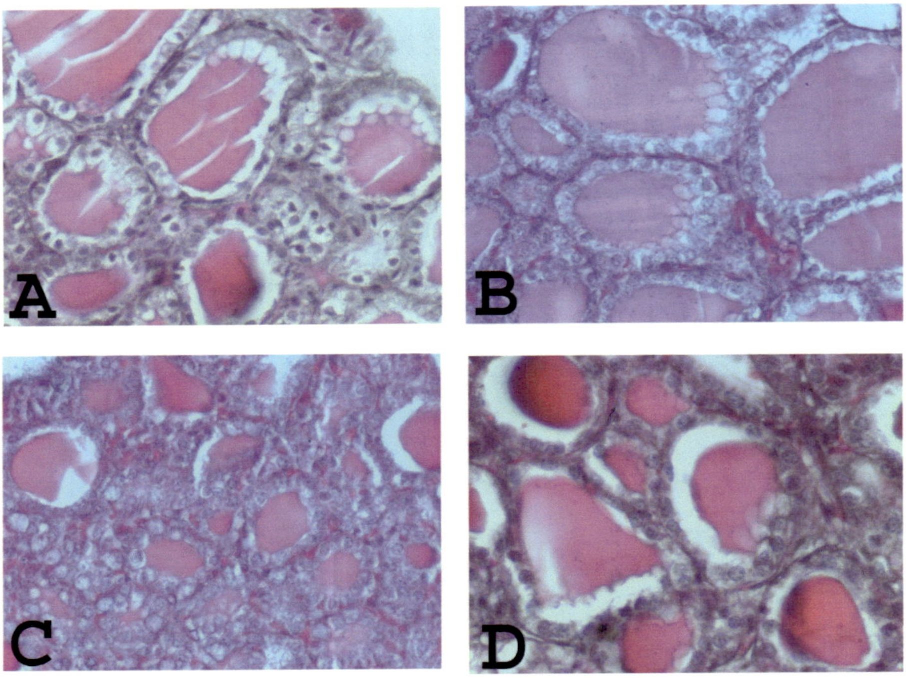

Figure 3.
Micrographs showing effects of melatonin on histology of thyroid in hypothyroid mice. Micrographs were taken at 40× objective of Olympus microscope BX-40. (A) control, (B) melatonin treated, (C) PTU treated, and (D) both melatonin and PTU treated.

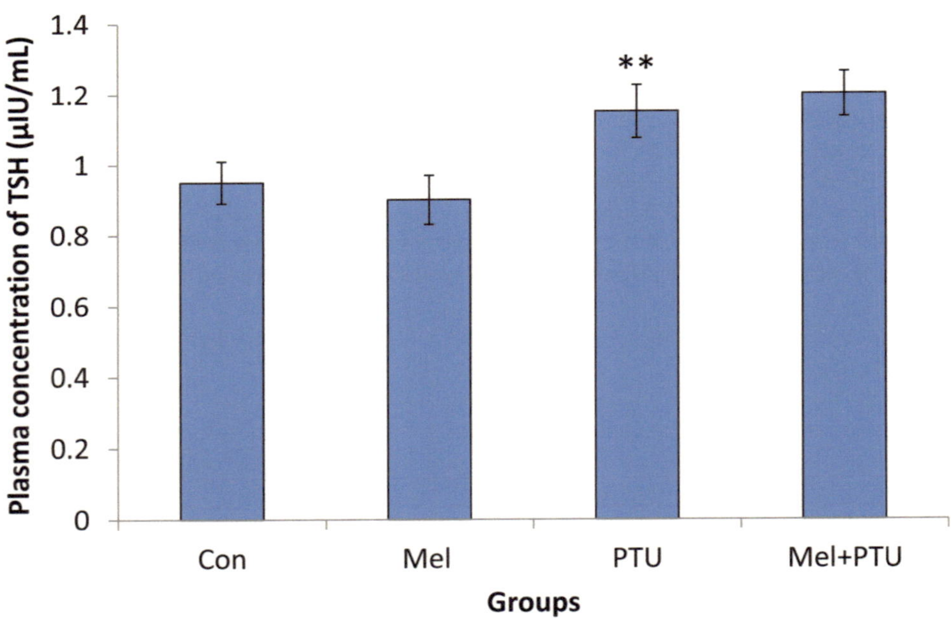

Figure 4.
Serum TSH concentration of experimental groups of mice. Histogram represents mean ± SEM. The mean differences were considered significant when $p < 0.01$. $^{**}p < 0.01$: Con vs. PTU.

thyroid gland (**Figures 6** and 7). PTU treatment caused a significant increase of MT1 and MT2 receptor proteins in the thyroid gland of mice in comparison with control mice. PTU caused stress in hypothyroid mice and induced the expression of

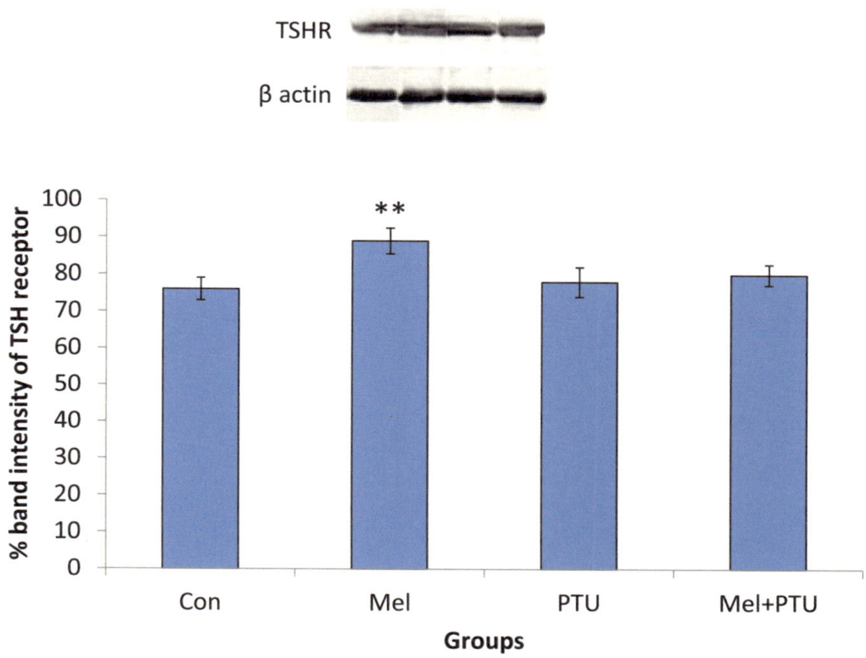

Figure 5.
Western blot analysis of TSH receptor protein expression in thyroid gland. β-actin was used as loading control. Lower panel shows percent expression of protein following Scion image analysis. Histogram represents mean ± SEM. The mean differences were considered significant when $p < 0.01$. $^{**}p < 0.01$: Con vs. Mel.

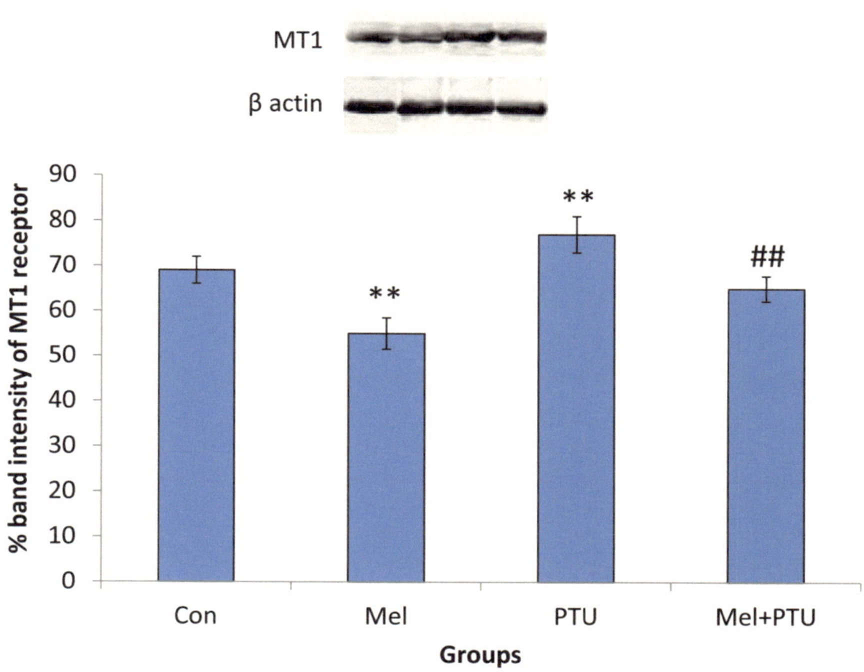

Figure 6.
Western blot analysis of MT1 receptor protein expression in thyroid gland. β-actin was used as loading control. Lower panel shows percent expression of protein following Scion image analysis. Histogram represents mean ± SEM. The mean differences were considered significant when $p < 0.01$. $^{**}p < 0.01$: Con vs. Mel; Con vs. PTU; $^{\#\#}p < 0.01$: PTU vs. Mel + PTU.

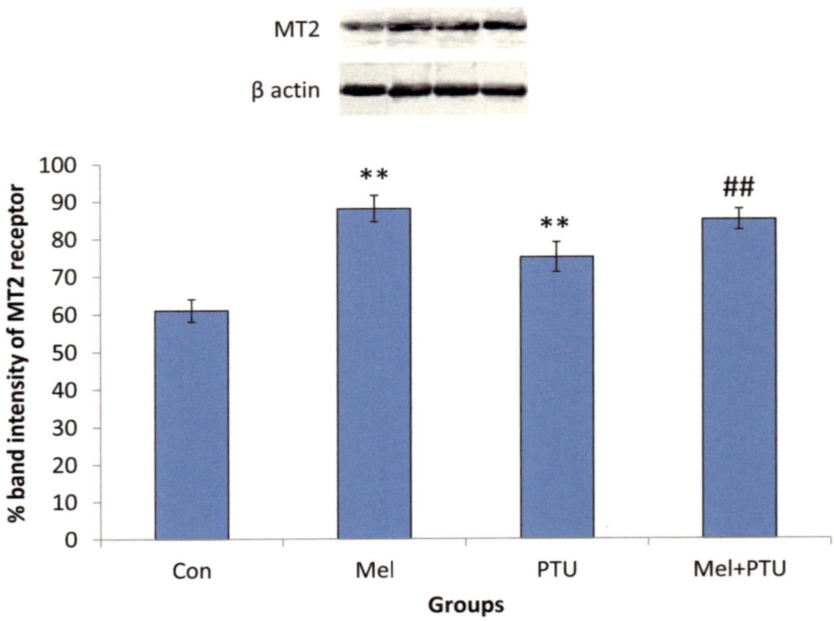

Figure 7.
Western blot analysis of MT2 receptor protein expression in thyroid gland. β-actin was used as loading control. Lower panel shows percent expression of protein following Scion image analysis. Histogram represents mean ± SEM. The mean differences were considered significant when $p < 0.01$. $^{**}p < 0.01$: Con vs. Mel; Con vs. PTU; $^{\#\#}p<0.01$: PTU vs Mel+PTU.

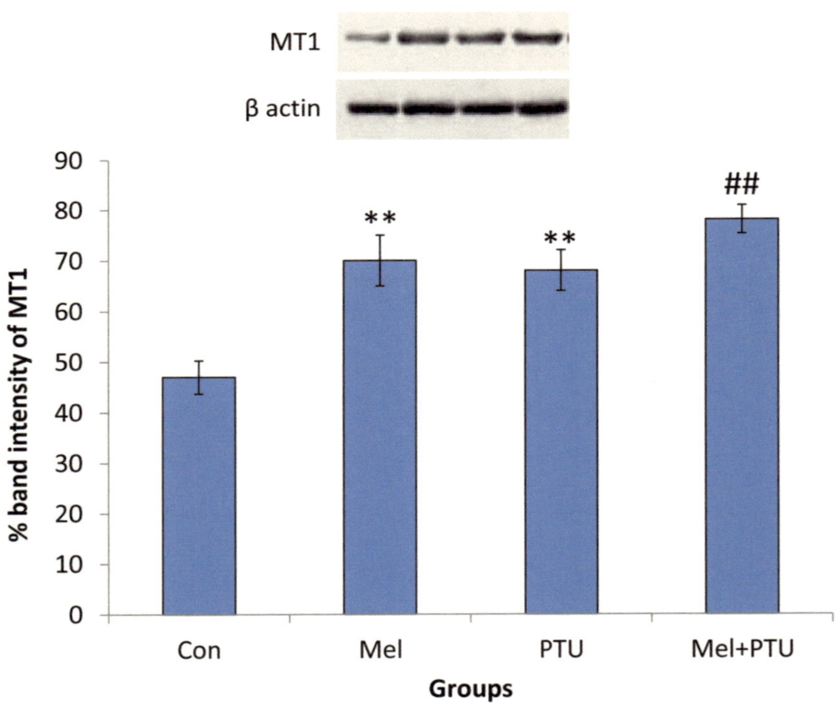

Figure 8.
Western blot analysis of MT1 receptor protein expression in pituitary gland. β-actin was used as loading control. Lower panel shows percent expression of protein following Scion image analysis. Histogram represents mean ± SEM. The mean differences were considered significant when $p < 0.01$. $^{**}p < 0.01$: Con vs. Mel; Con vs PTU; $^{\#\#}p<0.01$: PTU vs Mel+PTU.

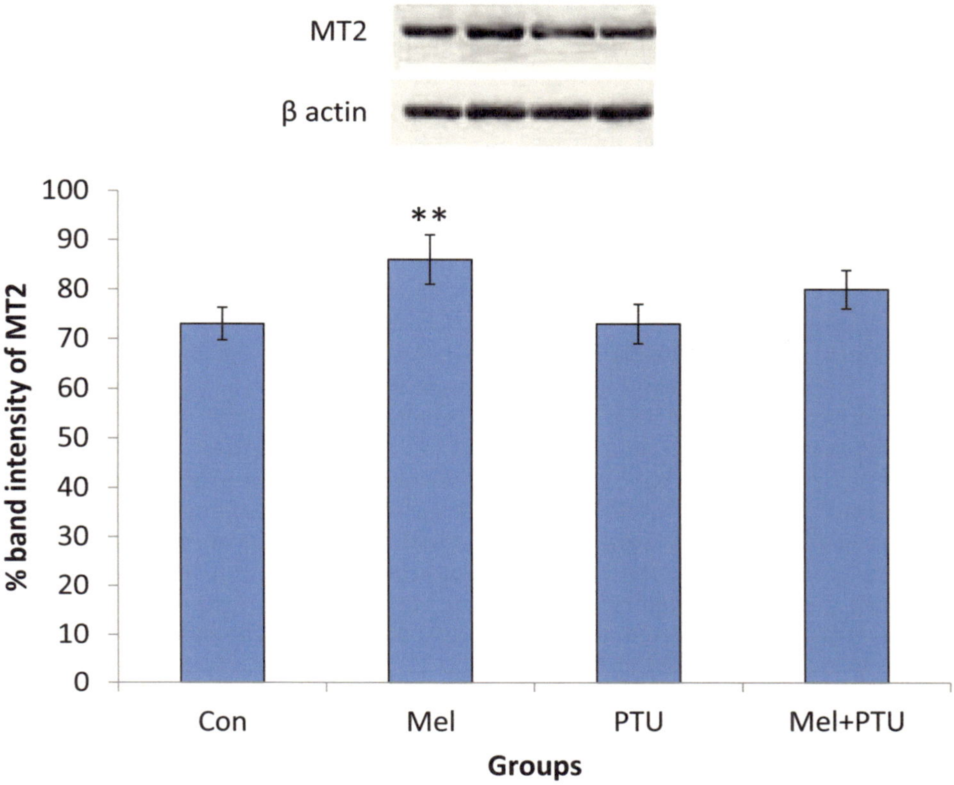

Figure 9.
Western blot analysis of MT2 receptor protein expression in pituitary gland. β-actin was used as loading control. Lower panel shows percent expression of protein following Scion image analysis. Histogram represents mean ± SEM. The mean differences were considered significant when $p < 0.01$. $^{**}p < 0.01$: Con vs. Mel.

MT1 and MT2 receptors in the thyroid of mice. Further, melatonin supplementation to hypothyroid mice caused increased expression of MT2 receptor proteins in comparison with hypothyroid mice.

3.5 Effect of melatonin on MT1 and MT2 receptor proteins in the pituitary gland

Melatonin supplementation increased the MT1 and MT2 receptor expression in the pituitary gland (**Figures 8** and **9**). Hypothyroid mice showed increased MT1 receptor protein expression, while MT2 receptor protein remained unaffected in comparison with control mice. Melatonin supplementation to hypothyroid mice caused a significant increase in MT1 receptor expression in the pituitary gland in comparison with the hypothyroid group. This result suggested that in the pituitary gland MT1 receptor is more responsive to melatonin in minimizing the PTU caused stress in hypothyroid mice.

4. Discussion

Metabolic suppression, lower respiration rate, and reduction in free radical formation reflect the hypothyroid state of an organism. In this study, we have noted a significant decrease in thyroid hormones level after melatonin treatment. Earlier workers reported that melatonin administration causes the impairment of thyroid function [20–22]. *In vitro* treatment of melatonin decreased the thyroid activity in a dose-dependent manner [23, 24]. Melatonin administration suppresses mitotic activity and so, strong inhibition of thyroid gland function was reported [8, 25, 26]. Treatment of 5-propyl-2-thiouracil (PTU) decreased the thyroid hormone levels as it is a known fact that antithyroid drugs cause a hypothyroid condition in mice. Melatonin-treated hypothyroid group showed an increased level of both T3 and T4 hormones. Melatonin treatment to hypothyroid mice counteracted the PTU caused suppression of both T3 and T4 hormone levels in the mice. Thakkar et al. [16] suggested that melatonin treatment reversed neonatal hypothyroidism-induced negative impacts on thyroid function.

Healthy mice showed a normal level of circulatory T_3 and T_4 levels and normal architecture of follicles in the thyroid gland. PTU treatment caused inhibition of thyroid hormonogenesis and thus reduced the production of T_4 and T_3 hormones. To fulfill the physiological demand, follicular colloid was excessively consumed and follicular size was reduced. Follicular cells enlarge in size with a small luminal area. The report suggested that to fulfill the hormonal demand follicular cells increase in size in PTU-treated rat [27]. Melatonin treatment minimized the PTU-induced harmful effects on hormonogenesis in thyroidal follicles and restored the follicular architecture in hypothyroid mice.

Serum TSH hormone level was unchanged, whereas TSH receptor expression in the thyroid gland increased after melatonin treatment. Reports suggested that the TSH hormone level was unaltered after melatonin administration [28]. PTU treatment increased the circulatory TSH hormone but TSH receptor expression on the thyroid gland was unaffected. Klecha et al. [29] documented the significant increase of TSH hormone level in experimentally induced hypothyroid mice. Melatonin treatment of hypothyroid mice increased the TSH hormone level, while TSH receptor proteins on the thyroid gland remained unaffected. Prolonged administration of melatonin to hypothyroid mice might be promoting thyroid function *via* increasing hypophysial TSH hormone secretion.

Administration of melatonin caused decreased MT1 melatonin receptor expression in the thyroid gland, whereas MT2 receptor expression in the thyroid gland increased. The report suggested that exogenous melatonin differentially influences the MT1 and MT2 receptor expression in the thyroid gland in an age-dependent manner [30]. PTU-induced hypothyroid condition caused increased expression of both MT1 and MT2 receptor proteins in thyroid gland. Melatonin treatment of hypothyroid mice caused increased MT2 receptor protein expression in thyroid gland. Prolonged treatment of melatonin in PTU-induced hypothyroid mice might be influencing thyroid function through activation of MT2 receptors in the thyroid gland.

Melatonin receptors are localized in most regions of the brain and also in the pituitary gland. (I^{125}) iodomelatonin binding assay suggested melatonin binding sites in the pituitary [31]. The melatonin receptor mRNA study also suggested that melatonin mediates its effects through MT1 and MT2 receptors in the pituitary gland. Exogenous melatonin caused an increase in MT1 and MT2 receptor protein expression in the pituitary gland. PTU caused the hypothyroid condition and induced the MT1 receptor protein expression in the pituitary gland of mice. Melatonin supplementation to hypothyroid mice caused a significant increase in MT1 receptor proteins expressed in the pituitary gland. This result suggested that the MT1 receptor of melatonin is more responsive to melatonin in the pituitary of hypothyroid mice. The report suggested the MT1 and MT2 receptor-mediated modulation of the pituitary function in laboratory mice [32].

5. Conclusion

The hypothalamohypophyseal and epithalamo-epiphyseal axes are the two important components of the integrated central neuroendocrine mechanism underlying the control of functional activity of the thyroid gland. In this study, melatonin treatment along with PTU treatment was effective in improving the thyroid function. Melatonin treatment of hypothyroid mice might improve the thyroid hormones *via* regulating the neuroendocrine axis and upregulation of hypophyseal TSH hormone. Exogenous melatonin differentially modulated the MT1 and MT2 receptor proteins expression in the pituitary and thyroid gland in hypothyroid experimental conditions. Therefore, the above findings may suggest that melatonin regulates the hypophyseal-thyroid function in hypothyroid mice through differential activation of MT1 and MT2 receptors in the pituitary and thyroid gland.

Acknowledgements

Financial support from the Council of Scientific and Industrial Research, New Delhi, and, University Grants Commission, DST-FIST, New Delhi, and help from the establishment of State Biotech Hub, Tripura University are gratefully acknowledged.

Conflict of interest

The authors declare that they have no conflict of interest that would prejudice the impartiality of this scientific work.

Author details

Shiv Shankar Singh*, Prashanjit Laskar, Anindita Deb and Sangita Sutradhar
Molecular Endocrinology Lab, Department of Zoology, Tripura University, Suryamaninagar, Tripura, India

*Address all correspondence to: shivssbhu@yahoo.co.in

References

[1] Mishra P, Samanta L. Oxidative stress and heart failure in altered thyroid States. Scientific World Journal. 2012;**2012**:741861. DOI: 10.1100/2012/741861

[2] Razvi S, Jabbar A, Pingitore A, Danzi S, Biondi B, Klein I, et al. Thyroid hormones and cardiovascular function and diseases. Journal of the American College of Cardiology. 2018;**71**:1781-1796

[3] Weitzel JM, Iwen KA, Seitz HJ. Regulation of mitochondrial biogenesis by thyroid hormone. Experimental Physiology. 2003;**88**:121-128

[4] Sahoo DK, Roy A, Chainy GBN. PTU-induced neonatal hypothyroidism modulates antioxidative status and population of rat testicular germ cells. National Academy Science Letters. 2006;**29**:133-135

[5] Porterfield SP, Hendrich CE. The role of thyroid hormones in prenatal and neonatal neurological development—Current perspectives. Endocrine Reviews. 1993;**14**:94-106

[6] Stagi S, Azzari C, Bindi G, Galluzzi F, Nanni S, Salti R. Undetectable serum IgA and low IgM concentration in children with congenital hypothyroidism. Clinical Immunology. 2005;**116**:94-98

[7] Nakamura R, Teshima R, Hachisuka A, Sato Y, Takagi K, Nakamura R, et al. Effects of developmental hypothyroidism induced by maternal administration of methimazole or propylthiouracil on the immune system of rats. International Immunopharmacology. 2007;**7**:1630-1638

[8] Sewerynek E, Wiktorska J, Lewinski A. Effects of melatonin on the oxidative stress induced by thyrotoxicosis in rats. Neuro Endocrinology Letters. 1999;**20**:157-161

[9] Brzezinska-Slebodzinska E. Fever induced oxidative stress: The effect on thyroid status and the 5′-monodeiodinase activity, protective role of selenium and vitamin E. Journal of Physiology and Pharmacology. 2001;**52**:275-284

[10] Nanda N. Oxidative stress in hypothyroidism. International Journal of Clinical and Experimental Physiology. 2016;**3**:4-9

[11] Ahmed OM, Ahmed RG, El-Gareibc AW, El-Bakry AM, El-Tawaba SM. Effects of experimentally induced maternal hypothyroidism and hyperthyroidism on the development of rat offspring: II-The developmental pattern of neurons in relation to oxidative stress and antioxidant defense system. International Journal of Developmental Neuroscience. 2012;**30**:517-537

[12] Reiter RJ, Tan DX, Cabrera J, D'Arpa D. Melatonin and tryptophan derivatives as free radical scavengers and antioxidants. Advances in Experimental Medicine and Biology. 1999;**467**:379-387

[13] Reiter RJ, Tan DX, Qi W, Manchester LC, Karbownik M, Calvo JR. Pharmacology and physiology of melatonin in the reduction of oxidative stress in vivo. Biological Signals and Receptors. 2000;**9**:160-171

[14] Rodriguez C, Mayo JC, Sainz RM, Antolin I, Herrera F, Martin V, et al. Regulation of antioxidant enzymes: A significant role for melatonin. Journal of Pineal Research. 2004;**36**:1-9

[15] Singh SS, Deb A. Sutradhar S. Effect of melatonin on arsenic-induced oxidative stress and expression of MT1 and MT2 receptors in the kidney of

laboratory mice. Biological Rhythm Research. 2020;**58**:1216-1230, DOI: 0.1080/09291016.2019.1566993

[16] Thakkar BP, Zala VM, Ramachandran AV. Simultaneous melatonin administration effectively deprograms the negative influence of neonatal hypothyroidism on immature follicles but not on mature follicles and body and ovarian weights. Journal of Endocrinology and Metabolism. 2011;**1**:220-226

[17] Klecha AJ, Genaro AM, Lysionek AE, Caro RA, Coluccia GA, Cremaschi GA. Experimental evidence pointing to the bidirectional interaction between the immune system and the thyroid axis. International Journal of Immunopharmacology. 2000;**22**:491-500

[18] Lowry OH, Rosebrough NJ, Farr AL, Randall RJ. Protein measurement with the Folin phenol reagent. The Journal of Biological Chemistry. 1951;**193**:265-275

[19] Singh SS, Deb A, Sutradhar S. Dexamethasone modulates melatonin MT2 receptor expression in splenic tissue and humoral immune response in mice. Biological Rhythm Research. 2017;**48**:425-435

[20] Zwirska-Korczala K, Kniazewski B, Ostrowska Z, Buntner B. Influence of melatonin on rat thyroid, adrenal and testis secretion during the day. Folia Histochemica et Cytobiologica. 1991;**29**:19-24

[21] Kniazewski B, Ostrowska Z, Zwirska-Korczala K, Bunter B. The influence of pinealectomy and single dose of melatonin administered at differ times of day on serum T3 and T4 concentrations in rats. Acta Physiologica Polonica. 1990;**41**:117-126

[22] Kniazewski B, Sobieraj H, Zwirska-Korczala K, Buntner B, Ostrowska Z. Influence of melatonin on thyroid secretion in pinealectomized rats. Endocrinologia Experimentalis. 1990;**24**:317-324

[23] Wright ML, Pikula A, Cykowski LJ, Kuliga K. Effect of melatonin on the anuran thyroid gland: Follicle cell proliferation, morphometry, and subsequent thyroid hormone secretion in vitro after melatonin treatment in vivo. General and Comparative Endocrinology. 1996;**103**:182-191

[24] Wright ML, Pikula A, Babski AM, Labieniec KE, Wolan RB. Effect of melatonin on the response of the thyroid to thyrotropin stimulation in vitro. General and Comparative Endocrinology. 1997;**108**:298-305

[25] Wajs E, Lewinski A. Inhibitory influence of late afternoon melatonin injections and the counter-inhibitory action of melatonin-containing pellets on thyroid growth process in male Wistar rats: Comparison with effects of other indole substances. Journal of Pineal Research. 1992;**13**:158-166

[26] D'Angelo G, Marseglia L, Manti S, Colavita L, Cuppari C, Impellizzeri P, et al. Atopy and autoimmune thyroid diseases: Melatonin can be useful? Italian Journal of Pediatrics. 2016;**42**:95

[27] Yi X, Yamamoto K, Shu L, Katoh R, Kawaoi A. Effect of propylthiouracil (PTU) administration on the synthesis and secretion of thyroglobulin in the rat thyroid gland: A quantitative immunoelectron microscopy study using immunogold technique. Endocrine Pathology. 1997;**8**(4): 315-325

[28] Siegrist C, Benedetti C, Orlando A. Lack of changes in serum prolactin, FSH, TSH, and estradiol after melatonin treatment in doses that improve sleep and reduce benzodiazepine consumption in sleep-disturbed, middle-aged, and elderly patients.

Journal of Pineal Research. 2001;**30**: 34-42

[29] Klecha AJ, Genaro AM, Gorelik G, Barreiro Arcos ML, Silberman DM, Schuman M, et al. Integrative study of hypothalamus–pituitary–thyroid–immune system interaction: Thyroid hormone-mediated modulation of lymphocyte activity through the protein kinase C signalling pathway. The Journal of Endocrinology. 2006;**189**:45-55

[30] Laskar P, Acharjee S, Singh SS. Effect of exogenous melatonin on thyroxine (T4), thyrotropin (TSH) hormone levels and expression patterns of melatonin receptor (MT1 and MT2) proteins on thyroid gland during different age groups of male and female Swiss albino mice. Advances in Bioresearch. 2015;**6**:7-14

[31] Williams LM, Hannah LT, Hastings MH, Maywood ES. Melatonin receptors in the rat brain and pituitary. Journal of Pineal Research. 1995;**19**: 173-177

[32] Laskar P, Singh SS. Receptor mediated action of melatonin in pituitary-thyroid-axis of lipopolysaccharide challenged mice. Annals of Thyroid Research. 2020;**6**(2):263-269

Section 2

Hypothyroidism: Treatment

Chapter 6

Hypothyroidism Therapy

Wissal Abassi, Nejmeddine Ouerghi and Anissa Bouassida

Abstract

Hypothyroidism refers to the common pathological disorder of thyroid hormone deficiency. The successful therapy for hypothyroidism is levothyroxine (LT4) administration, which is the same as thyroxine but produced synthetically. Serum thyrotropin (TSH) normalization with LT4 replacement therapy in hypothyroidism is generally needed to restore a euthyroid state. The daily dose of thyroxine therapy depends on various factors, such as body weight, age, and severity. It also differs from hypothyroidism during pregnancy to congenital hypothyroidism. The presence of various comorbidities may exist such as myxoedema coma, coronary artery disease, obesity, anemia and COVID-19 which necessitate individualized treatment. LT4 intolerance manifested with sympathetic hyperactivity may appear during the first hours after the LT4 administration. It requires starting with very low doses of LT4 that should be increased gradually, and reaching normal TSH may take several months. The sympathetic hyperactivity may be attributable to the presence of uncorrected iron-deficiency anemia that worsens by the use of thyroid hormone.

Keywords: Levothyroxine, dose, hypothyroidism, anemia, myxoedema coma, treatement

1. Introduction

Hypothyroidism refers to the common disorder of thyroid hormone deficiency. According to the time of onset, it may be present at birth (congenital) or develop later in life (acquired). Treatment of hypothyroidism consists of replacing the deficiency of thyroid hormone to improve symptoms and prevent the adverse consequences of hypothyroidism. Levothyroxine (LT4) that is identical to thyroxine but synthetically produced, is the most effective way to treat hypothyroidism. Treating hypothyroidism strategies are based on adopting an adequate dose of LT4, selecting a patient-appropriate serum thyrotropin (TSH) goal, and ensuring maintenance of that desired goal [1, 2]. The serum TSH normalization with LT4 replacement is generally needed to restore a euthyroid state. The daily LT4 dose must be individualized taking into account various factors such as body weight, age and severity of disease. Special situations may be coexisting requiring special treatement [2]. The purpose of this chapter is to provide the different therapeutic strategies of hypothyroidism management in various circumstances.

2. Congenital hypothyroidism

The guidelines of the American Academy of Pediatrics [3] and the European Society of Pediatric Endocrinology [4] recommends keeping TSH values below

Age	LT4 dose (lg/kg/day)
0–3 months	10–15
3–12 months	6–10
1–3 years	4–6
3–10 years	3–5
10–16 years	2–4
16 years	1.6
Modified from reference [1].	

Table 1.
Levothyroxine (LT4) weight-based dose in pediatric hypothyroidism.

5 μU/dl (optimally 0.5–2.0 μU/dl) for the first 3 years of life. LT4 is the treatment for hypothyroidism in children. Infants with suspected hypothyroidism require rapid evaluation and treatment, ideally within the first 2 weeks of life since delays in treatment of congenital hypothyroidism are correlated with poorer outcomes. Congenital hypothyroidism treatment should be initiated with 10–15 lg/kg of LT4 daily. Early starting treatment and adequate LT4 initial doses are associated with rapid normalization of thyroid function and improved neurodevelopmental outcomes [5].

Tablets might be crushed, suspended in a small amount of water, breast milk, or non–soy-based formula, and administered orally via a syringe. LT4 should not be administered with substances that may interfere with its absorption such as multivitamins containing calcium or iron, aluminum hydroxide and soy formula. The medication is administered once a day. The same dose should be repeated if there is immediate vomiting. If a dose is missed, it may be doubled the following day [6].

Serum thyroid function testing should be checked every 1–2 weeks until normal, and then every 1–2 months during the first year of life and every 2–4 months during the 2nd and 3rd years of life with an appropriate adjustment of LT4 dose [7]. The needed dose of LT4 to restore euthyroidism varied with the age and the hypothyroidism severity. The dose required per kilogram body mass to fully replace thyroid function is significantly higher in children than in adults and decreases with age (**Table 1**). Early and adequate prenatal treatment with LT4 prevents severe neurocognitive deficits and results in normal brain development [1].

3. Acquired hypothyroidism

The approach to treat acquired hypothyroidism is similar to that of congenital, consisting of replacing the deficiency of thyroid hormones to improve symptoms and prevent the adverse consequences of hypothyroidism. The target is to keep serum TSH <5 mIU/L (optimally 0.5–2 mIU/L) [8].

The recommended treatment is LT4 in tablets form administered once daily. Adherence to LT4 may be influenced by multiple factors such as the time of day when the medication is administered. Although the majority of experts recommend administration of LT4 prior to food consumption, but bedtime administration may be more convenient and does not appear to be associated with worse control of hypothyroidism in children and adolescents [9].

The dose of LT4 required to restore euthyroidism depends on patient age, body surface area, weight and severity of hypothyroidism (**Table 1**) [1]. The dose required to fully replace thyroid function is significantly higher in children than in adults and decreases with age. Thyroid function should be controlled 6 to 8 weeks after initiating therapy and then every 4 to 6 months until the child achieves final height or every 6 to 8 weeks following a change in LT4 dose [10].

4. Subclinical hypothyroidism

Subclinical hypothyroidism (SCH) is considered in two categories according to the elevation in serum TSH level: mildly increased TSH levels (4.0–10.0 mU/l), and more severely increased TSH value (>10 mU/l) [11]. For the American Thyroid Association recommendation, the goal of therapy is to normalize TSH levels within 0.5–3.5 mIU/L. The starting thyroid hormone treatment is recommended when the serum TSH is above 10 mIU/L. The treatment is generally not recommended when the TSH is 5–10 mIU/L except in patients with increased cardiovascular risk.

These guidelines suggest that LT4 is the treatment of choice with a daily dose of 25–75 mcg, depending on the degree of TSH elevation and to be adjusted based on clinical response and serum thyroid function test monitoring. Addition with liothyronine (T3) is not routinely recommended [1, 12].

For the European Thyroid Association, even in the absence of symptoms, replacement therapy with LT4 is recommended for younger patients (<65–70 years) who have serum TSH levels greater than 10 mIU/L and in younger SCH patients (serum TSH <10 mU/l) with symptoms suggestive of hypothyroidism. For older individuals (>80–85 years) with elevated serum TSH $\leq$ 10 mU/l, observation without hormonal treatment should be the strategy of choice. The aim is to reach a stable serum TSH in the lower half of the reference range (0.4–2.5 mU/l). A daily dose of LT4 between 50 and 100 μg for most SCH patients and between 25 and 50 mcg for those with cardiac disease and/or older age has been advised to normalize serum TSH. The use of T3 or combined LT4/T3 is no supported in the treatment [11].

According to the Latin American Thyroid Society, LT4 is started in individuals with a serum TSH greater than 10 mIU/L and considered to start in those with a serum TSH 4.5–10 mIU/L especially greater than 7 mIU/L, who are younger than 65 years with increased cardiovascular risk. Patients with persistent mild elevations in TSH with positive serum thyroid peroxidase (TPO) antibodies and ultrasound findings consistent with autoimmune thyroiditis could be considered for treatment. These guidelines recommends against treatment of elderly (65–80 years) patients with TSH levels less than 10 mIU/L [13].

The British Thyroid Association recommends starting treatment in patients with positive antibodies or serum TSH >10 mU/L. The guideline advise to start with LT4 doses between 50 and 125 mcg/day. Treatment should aim for TSH levels within the normal reference range. Older individuals or with cardiac disease, require smaller starting doses to avoid inducing cardiac ischaemia. Combined therapy with LT4 and liothyronine (LT3) is not routinely recommended [14].

The American Association of Clinical Endocrinology recommends starting treatment with LT4 in patients with TSH > 10 mIU / L or those with symptoms, cardiovascular risk factors or positive TPO antibody. The goal of LT4 therapy is to normalize TSH. The starting dose of LT4 is 1.5 mcg/kg in the absence of cardiovascular disease. In patients with cardiovascular disease, the starting dose of LT4 is 25 mcg and is up-titrated as needed [12]. The American Endocrine Society recommends against routine treatment of SCH patients with serum TSH levels of 4.5–10 mU/liter, but indicated that treatment was reasonable for patients with TSH levels greater than 10 mU/liter [15].

The American Association of Clinical Endocrinology recommends starting treatment with LT4 in patients with TSH > 10 mIU / L or those with symptoms, cardiovascular risk factors or positive TPO antibody. The goal of LT4 therapy is to normalize TSH. The starting dose of LT4 is 1.5 mcg/kg in the absence of cardiovascular disease. In patients with cardiovascular disease, the starting dose of LT4 is 25 mcg and is up-titrated as needed [12].

5. Myxoedema coma

Myxedema coma is the most extreme, life-threatening expression of severe hypothyroidism. Usual precipitating factors are discontinuation of therapy, infections and exposure to cold. Its clinical manifestations include hypothermia, respiratory depression, cardiovascular instability and altered mental status [1]. According to the American Thyroid Association guidelines, patients with myxedema coma should first receive empiric glucocorticoid coverage with intravenous glucocorticoid administration (at appropriate doses for the stressed state). These guidelines recommends a daily intravenous dose of 200 to 400 mcg of LT4, with lower doses given for patients who are of smaller stature, older, or who have a history of coronary disease or arrhythmia. Subsequently, daily dosing of 1.6 mcg/kg/day reduced to 75%, should be given.

Additional administration of intravenous T3 in a loading dose of 5–20 μg, followed by a maintenance dose of 2.5 to 10 mcg every 8 hours is recommended [1, 16–18]. For the Latin American Thyroid Society guidelines, LT4 replacement is the backbone of myxedema coma therapy. The daily starting dose is 300–500 μg/day followed by maintenance dose 50–100 μg/day. T3 can be added to therapy at 10–20 mg bolus followed by 10 μg every 4–6 hours [19]. The necessity of intravenous LT4 replacement is apparent, but administering LT4 alone or with a combination of LT4 and LT3 remains controversial [1, 16–18]. Carter et al. [20] prouved that combinated treatment with LT3 and LT4 are more beneficial than LT4 monotherapy to improve symptoms and to reverse the biochemical abnormalities in patients with myxedema coma. At the same Ono et al. [21] showed that patients receiving LT4 combined with LT3 had a lower mortality rate than those who received LT4 alone. T3 is an active hormone in the body with an immediate onset of action, whereas LT4 has a slow onset of action with relatively few adverse events. Also T3 affinity for the nuclear receptor is 10- to 20- fold higher than that of T4 and it reaches a peak level in 2–4 h after administration [22]. The beneficial effect of this combined treatment on neuropsychiatric symptoms has been confirmed because of the capacity of T3 to cross the blood brain barrier [23].

6. Pregnancy

6.1 Treatment of overt hypothyroidism in pregnancy

Women with overt hypothyroidism who contemplate pregnancy must first normalize TSH and thyroid hormone levels. LT4 is the first choice of treatment. American Thyroid Association guidelines specifies a goal of TSH less than 2·5 mIU/L in women planning to become pregnant [24]. Women with a previous diagnosis of hypothyroidism, should checked their serum TSH concentration and increased LT4 dose made as soon as possible after pregnancy is confirmed [25]. The LT4 replacement dose may be as high as 2.0–2.4 μg/kg body weight per day, which is 25–50% higher than levels used in the general population (1.6–1.8 μg/kg body weight) [26].

Once pregnant, women should increased the dose of LT4 by about 30–50%, beginning in the first 4–8 weeks of gestation and gradually increasing the dose through 16–20 weeks of gestation [27]. After initiation of therapy, thyroid function should be retested within 30–40 days, and then every 4–6 weeks. Maternal TSH concentrations should be maintained between 0·1–2·5 mIU/L in the first trimester, 0·2–3·0 mIU/L in the second, and 0·3–3·0 mIU/L in the third [27, 28].

6.2 Treatment of SCH in pregnancy

According to the American Thyroid Association guidelines, TSH levels should be keept below 2.5 mU/L and 3.0 mU/L in the first and second/third trimesters, respectively [28]. Autoantibodies to TPO should be mesured in women with SCH, since TPO positivity acts in synergy with SCH and it is an independent risk factor for pregnancy outcomes [29–31]. The rise of maternal TSH level increase the risk of miscarriage. This risk becomes even greater at a TSH level > 2.5 mU/L, accompanied by TPO positivity [24]. Pregnant women with SCH have a higher risk of several side effects such as pregnancy loss and premature birth [32]. In women receiving LT4 treatment for SCH, the risk of miscarriage in early pregnancy increases at a TSH level > 4.5 mU/L.

It was showed that LT4 treatment is capable to reduce the rate of pregnancy loss in TPO positive euthyroid women, therefore starting treatment with low doses of LT4 may be considered in TPO positive women with a history of recurrent pregnancy loss [33, 34]. Starting doses of LT4 were based on TSH levels, either 1 μg/kg/day (TSH 1.5–2.5 mU/L) or 0.5 μg/kg/day (TSH 0.5–1.5 mU/L), raising or lowering amounts by 0.5 μg/day at TSH levels >3 mU/L or < 0.5 mU/L, respectively [34].

7. Coronary artery disease

If untreated, hypothyroidism in patients with coronary heart disease might lead to ventricular arrhythmias, congestive heart failure or acute myocardial infarction.

Therefore, patients with coronary artery disease and hypothyroidism should be treated cautiously with thyroid hormone replacement [35]. Therapy is performed with the administration of LT4,that induced significant improvement in myocardial function, cardiac pump function and resting cardiac output [36]. However, in subjects with an already compromised myocardial blood supply due to coronary atherosclerosis, LT4 treatment may lead to anginal symptoms. A previous study showed that 2% among 1503 hypothyroid subjects presented new onset angina during LT4 therapy [37]. The recommended initial therapeutic dose for patients with pre-existing angina is 25 mg / day or even less and it should not be increased faster than at 4 week intervals [38].

8. Elderly

The serum TSH levels reference range is 4–5 mIU/L in the elderly patients. The hormone replacement with LT4 is the specific therapy for old individuals with hypothyroidism [39]. A normal starting dose of LT4 in an elderly subject is around 1 mg/kg/day, which is maintained for 4–6 weeks [40]. Dosage adjustments are guided by the TSH response and the clinical state, with emphasis on possible cardiac adverse effects [38]. Some experts recommended to increase the dosage by 25 μg in accordance with the patient's complaints [41]. While this therapeutic dose should be reduced of about 50 μg/day, or 25 μg/day when the patient was underweight or developed cardiovascular disease [39].

Hormone replacement with LT4 in patients with hypothyroidism requires specific therapy. LT4 is available in the form of tablets at various doses, but also in liquid form as an oral solution, thus enabling a customized dose titration [41]. The European Thyroid Association recommends treatment in patients above 70 years old who have a TSH >10 mUI/L and signs and/or symptoms of hypothyroidism [11]. However, the LT4 dose needs to be tailored, aiming for a TSH level between 4 and 10 mIU/L, while the patient's health condition and the potential presence of dyslipidemia and other metabolic derangements should be considered [42].

Likewise, van den Beld et al. [43] showed that low serum FT4 levels are associated with a longer 4-year survival, reflecting a possible adaptive mechanism to prevent excessive catabolism in the elderly. Hypothyroidism is prevalent among the elderly population, that's why efforts should be made to maintain optimal thyroid function with individualized treatment based on severity and comorbidities [43].

9. COVID-19

Hypothyroidism is not a risk factor associated with worse outcomes in COVID-19 positive patients, therefore no particular changes or consultations are envisaged relating to the diagnosis and treatment of hypothyroidism during the COVID-19 crisis [44]. It is recommended to pursue the same form, frequence and dosage of thyroid hormone replacement therapy. No particular therapeutic dosage was addressed. Regular blood test monitoring may be difficult, but when patients on thyroid hormone replacement feel significantly unwell or if there are significant weight changes, thyroid function testing with measurement of serum TSH and free thyroxine, is recommended to adjust medication if needed [45].

10. Obesity

LT4 is the treatment of patients developed SCH associated with hyperlipidae. T3 can be added for patients with adequately substituted hypothyroidism with obesity resistant to a lifestyle intervention or suspected of thyroid hormone conversion disorders [46].

An individual approach of treatment is necessary for obese patients with higher TSH levels. The clinical condition of elevated TSH without symptoms, thyroid antibodies, goiter, or associated thyroidal illness, was defined as obesity-associated hyperthyrotropinemia. The efficacy of thyroid hormone therapy in obese subjects with hyperthyrotropinemia has not yet been evaluated [47]. LT4 treatment of obese with hyperthyrotropinemia were performed only in children demonstrating that the increase TSH levels causes impaired glucose metabolism and dyslipidemia [48].

However, no evidence regarding a favorable effect of LT4 treatment on body weight in obese subjects with TSH < 10 mU/L and normal free thyroxine level has been demonstrated, so such treatment is not recommended. In such subjects dietary-behavioral intervention contributed to weight loss irrespective of LT4 use. However, in normal-weight patients with hypothyroidism LT4 treatment is an effective strategy to decrease total and LDL cholesterol, this effect is more pronounced in patients with TSH > 10 mU/L [11]. Obese individuals with isolated hyperthyrotropinemia without symptoms or other signs of thyroid disease should not be treated with thyroid hormone replacement [47].

The role of thyroid hormone in treating obesity was confirmed. So that T3 and T4 administration at varying doses and durations has been shown to enhance weight loss in obese euthyroid subjects [49]. Such therapy increased fat loss without decreasing skeletal muscle mass and strength or inducing cardiac dysfunction [50]. However, a systematic review by Kaptein et al. [51] describing the effects of T3 or T3/T4 treatment on weight loss in euthyroid individuals during caloric deprivation showed that T3 is associated with decreases in serum T4 concentrations, indicating pituitary suppression of TSH, resulting in subclinical hyperthyroidism.

11. Adrenal insufficiency

Glucocorticoid deficiency can accompany hypothyroidism and if it is not detected, it may be exacerbated by thyroid hormone replacement, raising the risk of adrenal crisis that can be fatal. The signs and symptoms of coexisting adrenal insufficiency are manifold and can be summarized as hypoglycemia, anemia, nausea, vomiting, alopecia areata, weight loss, abdominal pain, hypotension and hyperpigmentation [52]. If so, it is important to start with replacing glucocorticoids first before starting LT4 and then approaching LT4 replacement 5–7 days later. Starting by LT4 therapy can contribuate to an increased metabolism which raise demand of cortisol, leading then to an increased risk of an adrenal crisis [38, 53].

Not to be confused, the modest increase of serum TSH levels in cases of untreated adrenal insufficiency, might return to normal without for thyroid hormone replacement but only by the correct hydrocortisone replacement treatment. The diurnal variation in TSH levels is influenced by cortisol, it manifests higher concentrations at night and lower in the morning, which explains the increase in TSH levels in untreated adrenal insufficiency [54].

12. Differentiated thyroid cancer

Differentiated thyroid cancer should be treated with an appropriate expertise in order to ensure an optimal long-term treatment quality. The therapeutic approach is individualized and risk-adapted. Surgery and radioiodine therapy followed by LT4 substitution is the established therapeutic procedures. For widely invasive follicular thyroid carcinomas and follicular thyroid carcinoma with vascular infiltration, thyreoidectomy is recommended. Radioiodine therapy has been established for more than 60 years, consisted on systemic administration of radioiodine (I-131) to irradiate thyroid remnants as well as non-resectable or incompletely resected differentiated thyroid cancer.

The benefit of I-131 therapy was confirmed in individuals with differentiated thyroid cancer at high risk for recurrence, however in subjects with very low-risk differentiated thyroid cancer the positive effect of radioiodine on tumor-free and overall survival has not been proven [55]. Patients who undergone thyroidectomy for differentiated thyroid cancer, with or without additional treatment with I-131, need to take LT4 not only for treatment of hypothyroidism but also to minimize potential TSH stimulation of tumor growth [56]. The recommended levels of thyroid-stimulating hormone (mIU/L) targets in patients with differentiated thyroid cancer by American Thyroid Association are;<0.1 for high and intermediate risk (initial therapy) and persistent disease, 0.1–0.5 for high-risk disease free (follow-up) and low risk (initial therapy) and 0.3–2.0 for low-risk disease free (follow-up) [57].

13. Anemia

Anemia seems to be associated with thyroid dysfunction particularly hypothyroidism. Anemia was found in 65% of children and adolescents with hypothyroidism [58]. At the same, 10% of the individuals with thyroiditis manifested anemia. These patients may be particularly sensitive at the beginning of LT4 replacement therapy [59]. Lack of stimulation of erythroid colony development by thyroid hormones, reduction in oxygen distribution to tissues and diminution of erythropoietin level in the absence of thyroid hormones leads to anemia [60]. The correction of hypothyroidism promotes an adequate therapeutic response to iron salts. Iron may interfere with the absorption of the thyroid hormone, that's why LT4 should be taken at least four hours apart from the iron intake [52].

14. LT4 intolerance

A sympathetic hyperactivity may appear during the first hours after the LT4 administration manifested by precordialgia or palpitations. This condition requires starting with very low doses of LT4 that should be increased gradually, and reaching normal TSH may took several months. The sympathetic hyperactivity may be attributable to the presence of uncorrected iron-deficiency anemia that worsens by the use of thyroid hormone. The anemia should be corrected and thyroid hormone therapy should be stoped temporarily and then restarted at low doses. Occasionally, beta blockers can be used in these cases to control the symptoms during the first few weeks of thyroid replacement treatment [59, 61].

15. Conclusion

Hypothyroidism is a common disorder, diagnosed by the measurement of blood levels of thyroid hormones. In the face of this challenge, efforts should be made to maintain optimal thyroid function. Therapy of choise is the administration of LT4. Treatment should be individualized in accordance with the subject's age, weight, severity and comorbidities. Special situations can coexist such as adrenal insufficiency, pregnant women, elderly patients and patients with differentiated thyroid cancer, needing special considerations to ensure the patient's welfare and prevent therapeutic complications. Under- or over-treatment is common in clinical practice and should be avoided and lifelong follow-up is strongly indicated.

DOI: http://dx.doi.org/10.5772/intechopen.99978

Author details

Wissal Abassi[1,2]*, Nejmeddine Ouerghi[1,3] and Anissa Bouassida[1]

1 Research Unit, Sportive Performance and Physical Rehabilitation, High Institute of Sports and Physical Education of Kef, University of Jendouba, El Kef, Tunisia

2 Higher Institute of Sport and Physical Education of Ksar Said, University of "La Manouba", Manouba, Tunisia

3 University of Tunis El Manar, Faculty of Medicine of Tunis, Rabta Hospital, Tunis, Tunisia

*Address all correspondence to: wissalabassi93@gmail.com

References

[1] Jonklaas J, Bianco AC, Bauer AJ, Burman KD, Cappola AR, Celi FS, Cooper DS, Kim BW, Peeters RP, Rosenthal MS, Sawka AM. American Thyroid Association Task Force on Thyroid Hormone Replacement. Guidelines for the treatment of hypothyroidism: prepared by the american thyroid association task force on thyroid hormone replacement. Thyroid. 2014;24:1670-1751. DOI: 10.1089/thy.2014.0028.

[2] Jonklaas J. Update on the treatment of hypothyroidism. CurrOpin Oncol. 2016;28:18-25. DOI: 10.1097/CCO.0000 000000000242.

[3] American Academy of Pediatrics, Rose SR; Section on Endocrinology and Committee on Genetics, American Thyroid Association, Brown RS; Public Health Committee, Lawson Wilkins Pediatric Endocrine Society, Foley T, Kaplowitz PB, Kaye CI, Sundararajan S, Varma SK. Update of newborn screening and therapy for congenital hypothyroidism. Pediatrics. 2006 ; 117:2290-2303. DOI: 10.1542/ peds.2006-0915.

[4] European Society for Pediatric Endocrinology. Revised guidelines for neonatal screening programmes for primary congenital hypothyroidism. Horm Res. 1999;52:49-52. DOI: 10.1159/000023433.

[5] Rose SR, Brown RS, Foley T, Kaplowitz PB, Kaye CI, Sundararajan S, Varma SK. Update of newborn screening and therapy for congenital hypothyroidism. Pediatrics. 2006;117:2290-22303. DOI: 10.1542/ peds.2006-0915.

[6] Diaz A, Lipman Diaz EG. Hypothyroidism. Pediatr Rev. 2014;35:336-337. DOI: 10.1542/ pir.35-8-336.

[7] Léger J, Olivieri A, Donaldson M, Torresani T, Krude H, van Vliet G, Polak M, Butler G. Congenital Hypothyroidism Consensus Conference Group. European Society for Paediatric Endocrinology consensus guidelines on screening, diagnosis, and management of congenital hypothyroidism. Horm Res Paediatr. 2014;81:80-103. DOI: 10.1159/000358198.

[8] LaFranchi S. Acquired hypothyroidism in childhood and adolescence. In: Post TW, editor. UpToDate. Waltham. 2019.

[9] Akin O. Morning vs. bedtime levothyroxine administration: what is the ideal choice for children? J Pediatr Endocrinol Metab. 2018 ;31 : 1249-1255. DOI: 10.1515/jpem-2018-0168.

[10] Hanley P, Lord K, Bauer AJ. Thyroid Disorders in Children and Adolescents: A Review. JAMA Pediatr. 2016;170:1008-1019. DOI: 10.1001/jamapediatrics. 2016.0486.

[11] Pearce SH, Brabant G, Duntas LH, Monzani F, Peeters RP, Razvi S, Wemeau JL. 2013 ETA Guideline: Management of Subclinical Hypothyroidism. Eur Thyroid J. 2013 ; 2:215-228. DOI: 10.1159/000356507.

[12] Garber JR, Cobin RH, Gharib H, Hennessey JV, Klein I, Mechanick JI, Pessah-Pollack R, Singer PA, Woeber KA. Clinical practice guidelines for hypothyroidism in adults: cosponsored by the American Association of Clinical Endocrinologists and the American Thyroid Association. EndocrPract. 2012; 18:988-1028. DOI: 10.4158/EP12280.GL.

[13] Brenta G, Vaisman M, Sgarbi JA, Bergoglio LM, Andrada NC, Bravo PP, Orlandi AM, Graf H; Task Force on Hypothyroidism of the Latin American Thyroid Society (LATS). Clinical

practice guidelines for the management of hypothyroidism. Arq Bras Endocrinol Metabol. 2013;57:265-291. DOI: 10.1590/s0004-27302013000400003.

[14] Parretti H, Okosieme O, Vanderpump M. Current recommendations in the management of hypothyroidism: developed from a statement by the British Thyroid Association Executive. Br J Gen Pract. 2016;66:538-540. DOI:10.3399/bjgp16X687493.

[15] Gharib H, Tuttle RM, Baskin HJ, Fish LH, Singer PA, McDermott MT. Subclinical thyroid dysfunction: a joint statement on management from the American Association of Clinical Endocrinologists, the American Thyroid Association, and the Endocrine Society. J Clin Endocrinol Metab. 2005;90:581-585. DOI: 10.1210/jc.2004-1231.

[16] Dubbs SB, Spangler R. Hypothyroidism: causes, killers, and life-saving treatments. Emerg Med Clin North Am.2014; 32: 303-317. DOI: 10.1016/j.emc.2013.12.003.

[17] Wartofsky L. Myxedema coma. Endocrinol Metab Clin North Am.2006;35: 687-698. DOI: 10.1016/j.ecl.2006.09.003.

[18] Mathew V, Misgar RA, Ghosh S, Mukhopadhyay P, Roychowdhury P, Pandit K, Mukhopadhyay S, Chowdhury S. Myxedema coma: a new look into an old crisis. J Thyroid Res. 2011:493462. DOI: 10.4061/2011/493462.

[19] Dutta P, Bhansali A, Masoodi SR, Bhadada S, Sharma N, Rajput R. Predictors of outcome in myxoedema coma: a study from a tertiary care centre. Crit Care. 2008;12:R1. DOI: 10.1186/cc6211.

[20] Carter JN, Eastmen CJ, Corcoran JM, Lazarus L. Inhibition of conversion of thyroxine to triiodothyronine in patients with severe chronic illness. Clin Endocrinol (Oxf). 1976 ; 5: 587-594. DOI: 10.1111/j.1365-2265.1976.tb03861.x.

[21] Ono Y, Ono S, Yasunaga H, Matsui H, Fushimi K, Tanaka Y.Clinical characteristics and outcomes of myxedema coma: analysis of a national inpatient database in Japan. J Epidemiol.2017 ; 27: 117-122. DOI: 10.1016/j.je.2016.04.002.

[22] Biondi B, Wartofsky L. Combination treatment with T4 and T3: toward personalized replacement therapy in hypothyroidism? J Clin Endocrinol Metab.2012 ; 97: 2256– 2271. DOI: 10.1210/jc.2011-3399.

[23] Chernow B, Burman KD, Johnson DL, McGuire RA, O'Brian JT, Wartofsky L, Georges LP.T3 may be a better agent than T4 in the critically ill hypothyroid patient: evaluation of trans- port across the blood-brain barrier in a primate model. Crit Care Med.1983 ; 11: 99-104. DOI: 10.1097/00003246-198302000-00009.

[24] Alexander EK, Pearce EN, Brent GA, Brown RS, Chen H, Dosiou C, Grobman WA, Laurberg P, Lazarus JH, Mandel SJ, Peeters RP, Sullivan S. Guidelines of the American Thyroid Association for the Diagnosis and Management of Thyroid Disease During Pregnancy and the Postpartum. Thyroid. 2017;27:315-389. DOI: 10.1089/thy.2016.0457.

[25] Alexander EK, Marqusee E, Lawrence J, Jarolim P, Fischer GA, Larsen PR. Timing and magnitude of increases in levothyroxine requirements during pregnancy in women with hypothyroidism. N Engl J Med. 2004;351:241-249. DOI: 10.1056/NEJMoa040079.

[26] Abalovich M, Vázquez A, Alcaraz G, Kitaigrodsky A, Szuman G, Calabrese C, Astarita G, Frydman M, Gutiérrez S.

Adequate levothyroxine doses for the treatment of hypothyroidism newly discovered during pregnancy. Thyroid. 2013 ;23:1479-1483. DOI: 10.1089/ thy.2013.0024.

[27] De Groot L, Abalovich M, Alexander EK, Amino N, Barbour L, Cobin RH, Eastman CJ, Lazarus JH, Luton D, Mandel SJ, Mestman J, Rovet J, Sullivan S. Management of thyroid dysfunction during pregnancy and postpartum: an Endocrine Society clinical practice guideline. J Clin Endocrinol Metab. 2012;97:2543-2565. DOI: 10.1210/jc.2011-2803.

[28] Stagnaro-Green A, Abalovich M, Alexander E, Azizi F, Mestman J, Negro R, Nixon A, Pearce EN, Soldin OP, Sullivan S, Wiersinga W; American Thyroid Association Taskforce on Thyroid Disease During Pregnancy and Postpartum. Guidelines of the American Thyroid Association for the diagnosis and management of thyroid disease during pregnancy and postpartum. Thyroid. 2011;21:1081-1125. DOI: 10.1089/thy.2011.0087.

[29] Karakosta P, Alegakis D, Georgiou V, Roumeliotaki T, Fthenou E, Vassilaki M, Boumpas D, Castanas E, Kogevinas M, Chatzi L. Thyroid dysfunction and autoantibodies in early pregnancy are associated with increased risk of gestational diabetes and adverse birth outcomes. J Clin Endocrinol Metab. 2012;97:4464-4472. DOI: 10.1210/ jc.2012-2540.

[30] Liu H, Shan Z, Li C, Mao J, Xie X, Wang W, Fan C, Wang H, Zhang H, Han C, Wang X, Liu X, Fan Y, Bao S, Teng W. Maternal subclinical hypothyroidism, thyroid autoimmunity, and the risk of miscarriage: a prospective cohort study. Thyroid. 2014 ;24:1642-1649. DOI: 10.1089/ thy.2014.0029.

[31] Ying H, Tang YP, Bao YR, Su XJ, Cai X, Li YH, Wang DF. Maternal TSH level and TPOAb status in early pregnancy and their relationship to the risk of gestational diabetes mellitus. Endocrine. 2016;54:742-750. DOI: 10.1007/s12020-016-1022-6.

[32] Maraka S, Ospina NM, O'Keeffe DT, Espinosa De Ycaza AE, Gionfriddo MR, Erwin PJ, Coddington CC 3rd, Stan MN, Murad MH, Montori VM. Subclinical Hypothyroidism in Pregnancy: A Systematic Review and Meta-Analysis. Thyroid. 2016;26:580-590. DOI: 10.1089/thy.2015.0418.

[33] Lepoutre T, Debieve F, Gruson D, Daumerie C. Reduction of miscarriages through universal screening and treatment of thyroid autoimmune diseases. Gynecologic and obstetric investigation.2012 ; 74 : 265-273. DOI:10.1159/000343759.

[34] Negro R, Formoso G, Mangieri T, Pezzarossa A, Dazzi D, Hassan H. Levothyroxine treatment in euthyroid pregnant women with autoimmune thyroid disease: effects on obstetrical complications. J Clin Endocrinol Metab. 2006 ;91:2587-2591. DOI: 10.1210/ jc.2005-1603.

[35] Aronow WS. The heart and thyroid disease. Clin Geriatr Med. 1995;11:219-229.

[36] Mourouzis I, Forini F, Pantos C, Iervasi G. Thyroid hormone and cardiac disease: from basic concepts to clinical application. J Thyroid Res. 2011;2011:958626. DOI: 10.4061/2011/ 958626.

[37] Keating FR, Parkin TW, Selby JB, Dickinson LS. Treatment of heart disease associated with myxedema. Prog Cardiovasc Dis. 1961; 3: 364-381. DOI: 10.1016/s0033-0620(61)90004-4

[38] Khandelwal D, Tandon N. Overt and subclinical hypothyroidism: who to treat and how. Drugs. 2012; 72:17-33. DOI: 10.2165/11598070-000000000-00000.

[39] Cooper DS. Thyroid disease in the oldest old: the exception to the rule. JAMA. 2004;292:2651-2654. DOI: 10.1001/jama.292.21.2651.

[40] Laurberg P, Andersen S, Bülow Pedersen I, Carlé A. Hypothyroidism in the elderly: pathophysiology, diagnosis and treatment. Drugs Aging. 2005;22:23-38. DOI: 10.2165/00002512-200522010-00002.

[41] Duntas LH, Yen PM. Diagnosis and treatment of hypothyroidism in the elderly. Endocrine. 2019;66:63-69. DOI: 10.1007/s12020-019-02067-9.

[42] Jonklaas J, Razvi S. Reference intervals in the diagnosis of thyroid dysfunction: treating patients not numbers. Lancet Diabetes Endocrinol. 2019;7:473-483. DOI: 10.1016/S2213-8587(18)30371-1.

[43] Van den Beld AW, Visser TJ, Feelders RA, Grobbee DE, Lamberts SW. Thyroid hormone concentrations, disease, physical function, and mortality in elderly men. J Clin Endocrinol Metab. 2005;90: 6403-6409. DOI: 10.1210/jc.2005-0872.

[44] Chaker L, Bianco AC, Jonklaas J, Peeters RP. Hypothyroidism. Lancet. 2017;390:1550-1562. DOI: 10.1016/S0140-6736(17)30703-1.

[45] Boelaert K, Visser WE, Taylor PN, Moran C, Léger J, Persani L. ENDOCRINOLOGY IN THE TIME OF COVID-19: Management of hyperthyroidism and hypothyroidism. Eur J Endocrinol. 2020;183:G33-G39. DOI: 10.1530/EJE-20-0445.

[46] Krotkiewski M. Thyroid hormones in the pathogenesis and treatment of obesity. Eur J Pharmacol. 2002; 440: 85-98. DOI: 10.1016/s0014-2999(02)01420-6.

[47] Gajda SN, Kuryłowicz A, Żach M, Bednarczuk T, Wyleżoł M. Diagnosis and treatment of thyroid disorders in obese patients - what do we know? Endokrynol Pol. 2019;70:271-276. DOI: 10.5603/EP.a2018.0089.

[48] Radhakishun NN, van Vliet M, von Rosenstiel IA, Weijer O, Beijnen JH, Brandjes DP, Diamant M. Increasing thyroid-stimulating hormone is associated with impaired glucose metabolism in euthyroid obese children and adolescents. J Pediatr Endocrinol Metab. 2013;26:531-537. DOI: 10.1515/jpem-2012-0302.

[49] Adler SM, Wartofsky L.The nonthyroidal illness syndrome. Endocrinol Metab Clin North Am. 2007 ; 36:657– 672. DOI: 10.1016/j.ecl.2007.04.007.

[50] Burman KD, Wartofsky L, Dinterman RE, Kesler P, Wannemacher RW Jr. The effect of T3 and reverse T3 administration on muscle protein catabolism during fasting as measured by 3-methylhistidine excretion. Metabolism. 1979;28:805-813. DOI: 10.1016/0026-0495(79)90206-3.

[51] Kaptein EM, Beale E, Chan LS. Thyroid hormone therapy for obesity and nonthyroidal illnesses: a systematic review. J Clin Endocrinol Metab. 2009;94:3663-3675. DOI: 10.1210/jc.2009-0899.

[52] Rizzo LFL, Mana DL. Treatment of hypothyroidism in special situations. Medicina (B Aires). 2020;80:83-93.

[53] Arima H, Iwama S, Inaba H, Ariyasu H, Makita N, Otsuki M, Kageyama K, Imagawa A, Akamizu T. Management of immune-related adverse events in endocrine organs induced by immune checkpoint inhibitors: clinical guidelines of the Japan Endocrine Society. Endocr J. 2019;66:581-586. DOI: 10.1507/endocrj.EJ19-0163.

[54] Samuels MH. Effects of variations in physiological cortisol levels on

thyrotropin secretion in subjects with adrenal insufficiency: a clinical research center study. J Clin Endocrinol Metab 2000; 85: 1388-1393. DOI:10.1210/jcem.85.4.6540

[55] Schmidbauer B, Menhart K, Hellwig D, Grosse J. Differentiated Thyroid Cancer-Treatment: State of the Art. Int J Mol Sci. 2017;18:1292. DOI: 10.3390/ijms18061292.

[56] McGriff NJ, Csako G, Gourgiotis L, Lori C G, Pucino F, Sarlis NJ. Effects of thyroid hormone suppression therapy on adverse clinical outcomes in thyroid cancer. Ann Med. 2002;34:554-564. DOI: 10.1080/078538902321117760.

[57] Cooper DS, Doherty GM, Haugen BR, Kloos RT, Lee SL, Mandel SJ, Mazzaferri EL, McIver B, Pacini F, Schlumberger M, Sherman SI, Steward DL, Tuttle RM. American Thyroid Association (ATA) Guidelines Taskforce on Thyroid Nodules and Differentiated Thyroid Cancer, Revised American Thyroid Association management guidelines for patients with thyroid nodules and differentiated thyroid cancer. Thyroid. 2009;19:1167-1214. DOI: 10.1089/thy.2009.0110.

[58] Chu JY, Monteleone JA, Peden VH, Graviss ER, Vernava AM. Anemia in children and adolescents with hypothyroidism. Clin Pediatr (Phila). 1981; 20:696-699. DOI: 10.1177/000992288102001102.

[59] Cinemre H, Bilir C, Gokosmanoglu F, Bahcebasi T. Hematologic effects of levothyroxine in iron-deficient subclinical hypothyroid patients: a randomized, double-blind, controlled study. J Clin Endocrinol Metab. 2009;94:151-156. DOI: 10.1210/jc.2008-1440.

[60] Soliman AT, De Sanctis V, Yassin M, Wagdy M, Soliman N. Chronic anemia and thyroid function. Acta Biomed. 2017 28;88:119-127. DOI: 10.23750/abm.v88i1.6048.

[61] Roberts CG, Ladenson PW. Hypothyroidism. Lancet. 2004;363:793-803. DOI: 10.1016/S0140-6736(04)15696-1.

Section 3

Hypothyroidism: Health Implications

Chapter 7

Cytokine Storm in Hypothyroidism in Infertile Women

Neha Sharma, Sanghapriya Mukherjee and Aparajita Kushwaha

Abstract

Thyroid dysfunction interferes with several aspects of reproduction along with pregnancy. Hypothyroidism in females leads to an elevated level of hormone prolactin which decreases levels of follicle-stimulating hormone (FSH), luteinizing hormone (LH) and finally causes infertility. Obesity acts upon the reproductive cycle by decreasing oestrogen metabolism stimulating menstrual disturbance along with an ovulation. But till date, one of the most underestimated obstacles in fertility is inflammation. Hypothyroidism leads to inflammation in secondary epithelial cells of thyroid gland. This affects immune, nervous system and endocrinal functions of body. Inflammation contributes to oestrogen dominance, a hormonal state that consists of having too little progesterone in the body compared to oestrogen. This leads to progesterone resistance, prevention of progesterone hormone receptors from working properly. This condition also leads to infertility in hypothyroid females. Therefore, not only hormonal profile is sufficient to check up for reproductive problems in the female, but also inflammatory markers like IL-6 and CRP should be added to this profile.

Keywords: hypothyroid, cytokine storm, infertility, inflammation, inflammatory markers

1. Introduction

The risk of facing thyroid problems is nearly 10 times higher for women than for men. For the normal functioning of the ovaries and maturation of eggs, there is a correlation between reproductive hormones (oestrogen and progesterone) and thyroid hormones in females [1]. The balancing of thyroid hormones is thus essential for fertility in women (**Figure 1**). The function of reproductive hormones can be altered by hyper- or hypo-secretion of thyroid hormones and result in thyroid-related infertility [2].

Apart from thyroid hormone imbalance, infertility has a lot to do with the lifestyle of a woman. Hormones released by the thyroid gland can have a variety of effects on the reproductive systems like delay or early onset of puberty, amenorrhea, ovulation, miscarriage, premature birth, etc. Smoking, drinking, stress, consumption of fast food, depression, delayed conception and age are some of the other factors responsible for infertility.

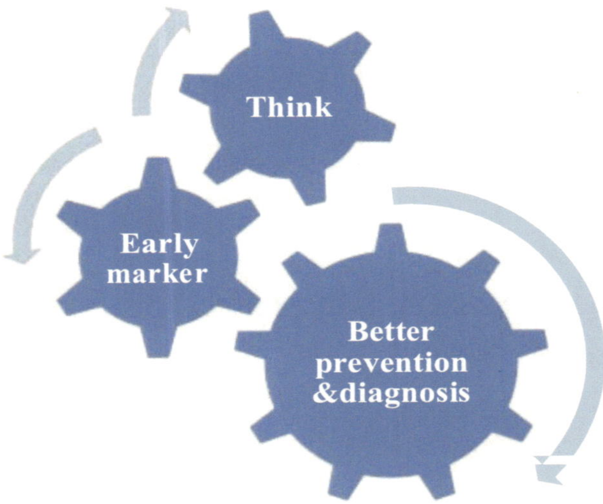

Figure 1.
Outline diagram for awareness. (Courtesy: Dr. Neha Sharma).

2. Hormonal regulation of menstrual cycle: oestrogen and progesterone

In females, usually most oestrogen and progesterone are released by ovarian follicles and corpus luteum, and by placenta at the time of pregnancy. The secretion reaches its peak in 7 days after ovulation and then declines if conception and implantation occur. Two types of oestrogen are produced: oestradiol and oestrone. Small amounts of oestrogen are produced by cells of corona radiata, theca interna and corpus luteum [3].

The main role of oestrogen is endometrial growth, follicle development or ovulation, increased proliferation of epithelial cells in vagina and uterus, stimulation of synthesis of proteins like contractile proteins in myometrial muscle fibres [3].

Other functions of oestrogen include promoting endometrial growth, increasing bone formation, increasing hepatic synthesis of binding proteins, increasing level of circulating coagulation factors II, VIII, IX, X, III and plasminogen and increasing adhesiveness of platelets.

Functions of progesterone are:

- It stimulates the secretary activity of uterine tubes, uterus and the vagina. This is responsible for pre-gestational changes in endometrium and along with oestrogen, it is responsible for the cyclic changes in cervix and vagina.

- Increases membrane potential of myometrial fibres.

Oestradiol as well as progesterone both act on the endometrium: Oestradiol promotes the growth of constituents of the endometrium, while progesterone helps to change from a proliferative pattern into a secondary pattern. When the levels of oestrogen and progesterone fall, it leads to the end of the cycle as endometrium cannot be maintained further, and as a result menstruation occurs [4].

3. Gonadotropin releasing hormones (GnRH)

GnRH activates a surge of LH preceding ovulation [3]. Hypothalamic GnRH is released in an exciting manner by caudate nucleus of hypothalamus. GnRH production is acted upon by oestradiol or catecholamine neurotransmitters. It reaches to anterior pituitary by hypothalamo-pituitary portal plexus.

Function of GnRH:

- Ovarian follicles act in response to pituitary gonadotrophin secretion by producing the main ovarian hormone oestradiol and progesterone.
- The production of LH and FSH from pituitary is caused by pulses of GnRH, which is produced by hypothalamus.

3.1 Prolactin

Prolactin is secreted through cells of adenohypophysis. The main function of prolactin is the initiation and maintenance of lactation. For ductal growth and development of breasts, prolactin is a must. This is required for synthesis of specific milk proteins (casein, gamma lactalbumin). Although the exact intracellular mechanism of prolactin action is yet not known, prolactin regulates transport of lipoproteins in adrenal gland, testis and ovary to ensure the continuous supply of LDL for steroid genesis. It also promotes synthesis of enzymes of androgen pathway, which facilitates the conversion of pregnenolone to dehydroepiandrosterone and/or dehydroepiandrosterone sulphate [5].

Release of prolactin is under a tonal inhibitory control through hypothalamus. This is also influenced through:

a. Oestradiol: Ovarian oestradiol augments prolactin secretion or action is responsible for the difference in concentrations of prolactin in adult, pre-pubertal or menopausal women)

b. Sleep: Moderate rise in prolactin concentrations at the time of sleep is seen.

c. Stress: Various types of stress, e.g., physical aggression, cold, surgery and heat are all known to raise prolactin levels.

d. Pharmacological agents: Tranquillisers may obstruct dopaminergic receptors, for example the phenothiazine derivatives, or slow down dopamine reuptake from inter-neuronal cleft, for example the tricyclic depressants [6]

Hyperprolactinemia is the most common in hypothalamic–pituitary disorder found in clinical endocrinology [1]. PRL concentration is also increased in women who have a problem in fertility like anovulation, with or without menstrual irregularity, amenorrhea and galactorrhoea. Causes of hyperprolactinemia include:

a. The presence of a prolactin-producing adenoma.

b. Tumour of the pituitary gland, which obstructs the inhibitory control of the hypothalamus.

c. In a few endocrine diseases such as primary hypothyroidism, anti-hypertensive polycystic ovarian syndrome.

d. Intake of antidepressants.

Hyperprolactinemia can interrupt ovarian physiology at various levels, including steroidogenesis, follicular maturation and ovulation, the process of luteinisation and corpus luteum function [7].

3.2 LH and FSH

The gonadotrophins FSH and LH are hormones that are protein in nature secreted by anterior pituitary [1]. LH and FSH are glycoproteins as they are made up of two peptide chains, alpha and specific beta subunit. Both hormones are glycosylated, which determines their bioactivity and half-life.

Secretion of gonadotrophins, LH, FSH is controlled by luliberin. This stimulates the emission of LH effectively than follitropin production, plasma levels of sex

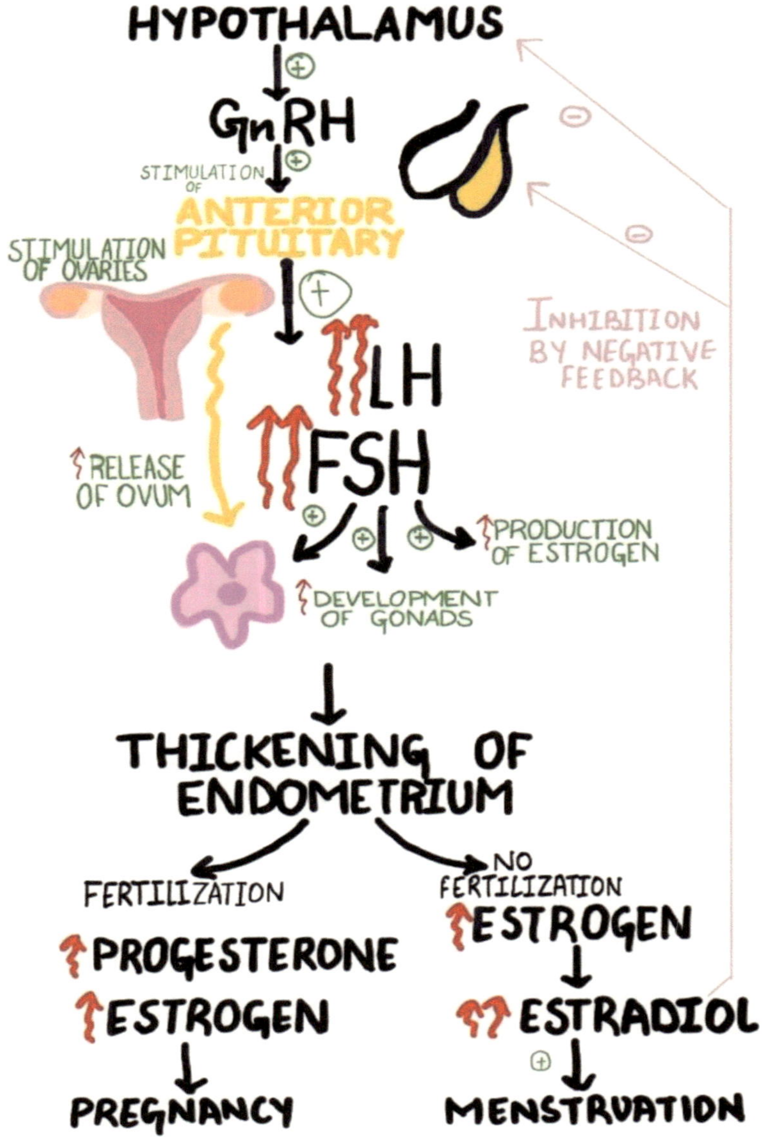

Figure 2.
Hormonal regulation of menstrual cycle. (Courtesy- Ms. Aparajita Kushwaha, Ms. Sanghapriya Mukherjee).

hormone by positive and negative feedback. It is also controlled by hormone Inhibin, which is produced by the Graafian follicles [3].

FSH and LH work on gonads to trigger gametogenesis and synthesis of hormones associated with it. At the follicular stage, FSH and LH trigger oestrogen production by the developing follicle.

LH and FSH have significant actions on the ovary:

a. The major effect of FSH is to trigger growth and development of Graafian follicles, while on the other hand, LH leads to ovulation.

b. Ovarian steroids are produced by actions on FSH and LH.

When Graafian follicle enlarges, it increases the amount of oestrogen and oestradiol production. Within mid-cycle, surge of LH is seen, so ovulation takes place and the Graafian follicle is changed into corpus luteum by progesterone activity [4].

FSH also reaches its peak at the end of the follicular stages, a part of the surge of pre-ovulatory gonadotrophin (**Figure 2**) [6].

4. Thyroid stimulating hormone (TSH)

The thyroid stimulating hormone, also called thyrotropin, is secreted from adenohypophysis in reaction to thyroid releasing hormone (TRH). It is a glycoprotein in nature, containing 209 amino acids [3]. It is chiefly associated with the growth of thyroid gland and stimulation of its hormonal activity [5].

Functions of TSH.

1. It has a wide range of activity on the follicular cells:

    a. TSH acts directly on the thyroid gland to raise the secretion of thyroid hormones and help in formation of follicular cells (cuboidal and columnar shaped).

    b. Increase the number of follicular cells, also known as hyperplasia.

    c. TSH decreases the volume of follicular colloid, thereby increasing vascularity of the gland.

    d. Other effects of TSH on follicular cell activity include:

        - Increases oxygen consumption.

        - Increased glucose utilisation.

        - Increased carbon dioxide production.

        - Increased formation of phospholipids.

        - Increased synthesis of RNA and protein [8, 9].

2. TSH stimulation leads to the secretion of the stored thyroid hormone from the follicular colloid.

3. TSH promotes the production of thyroid hormone by increasing the transportation of iodine into the follicular cells or by enhancing organic

binding of iodine to thyroxine as well as subsequent coupling to form thyroid hormone on the surface of thyroglobulin molecules [10].

4. TSH along with T3 and T4 plays an important role in regulation, synthesis, development, metabolism and overall growth of the body. The functions include:

    a. Strengthening metabolism of carbohydrates, proteins and lipids.

    b. Reinforcement of growth and development.

    c. Regulation and transportation of water and electrolytes.

    d. Stimulation of the cardiovascular system.

    e. Stimulation of the Central Nervous System [11].

5. Hypothyroidism

Hypothyroidism is a condition characterised by elevated serum thyroid stimulating hormone level and decreased serum levels of T3 and T4 due to under activity of the thyroid gland. According to NHANES (National Health and Nutrition Examination Survey), in the last 6 years, the prevalence of hypothyroidism is 4.6% [12]. Thyroid disorders, hypothyroidism or hyperthyroidism are more common in females than in males.

5.1 Causes of hypothyroidism

The causes of hypothyroidism are divided into six categories:

- Hypothyroidism through compensatory thyroid enlargement owing to transient and progressive destruction by hormone biosynthesis, for example, goitrous hypothyroidism.

- Permanent loss and atrophy of tissue of thyroid gland, for example atrophic thyroidism.

- Transient Hypothyroidism, i.e., transient deficiency of thyroid hormones a few days prior to birth.

- Central hypothyroidism due to insufficient stimulation of thyroid gland as a result of hypothalamic or pituitary disease.

- Resistance to thyroid hormone (RTH), which is a deficiency of thyroid hormone [13].

Symptoms of hypothyroidism include cold intolerance, fatigue, lethargy, decreased metabolism, weight gain, brittle nails and dry skin.

5.2 Consequences of hypothyroidism

Thyroid disease is associated with a wide range of metabolic abnormalities, owing to the fact that thyroid hormones act on majority of the metabolic pathways.

6. Infertility

What is infertility?

Infertility is defined as an inability to conceive after 1 year of regular intercourse without contraception. WHO defined infertility as 'a disease of the reproductive system which is explained by inability to achieve pregnancy after twelve months or more of regular unprotected intercourse' [14].

6.1 Types of infertility

First degree or primary infertility.

When a couple is not able to conceive even having unprotected intercourse over a period of minimum 1 year, it is defined as the first degree or primary infertility [15].

Second degree or secondary infertility.

Secondary infertility occurs when a couple cannot conceive for the second time even after regular intercourse without any contraceptives. To count as secondary infertility, the first childbirth should not have occurred with the help of any kind of fertility medication or procedures like IVF [15].

6.2 Causes of infertility

Problems of infertility start from hormonal dysfunction of the hypothalamic pituitary gonadal axis. The major cause of infertility is a disorder of oocyte production, ovulation, healthy sperm production, fallopian tube dysfunction, and lastly, improper implantation of the embryo in the uterine wall.

Sexually transmitted diseases like gonorrhoea and syphilis may also lead to infertility.

PCOD, obesity, thyroid issues and imbalanced hormones of the menstrual cycle can also lead to infertility through a surge in the cytokine levels of the body (cytokine storm).

Multiple studies show that cigarette smoking, narcotics and drugs have been established to impair fertility in both males and females (**Figure 3**). Smoking has unfavourable effects on tubal function, secretion of hormones and cervical mucus production [16].

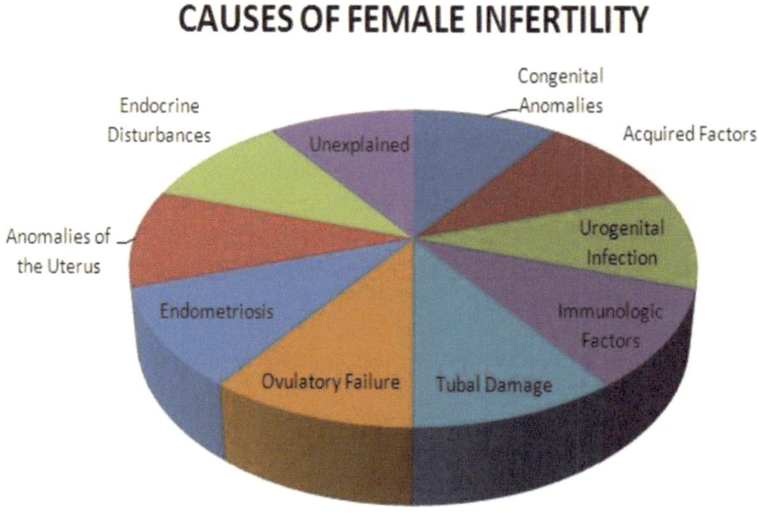

Figure 3.
Causes of infertility (Courtesy – Dr. Neha Sharma).

Ingestion of alcohol has also been shown as a reason to decrease gonadotrophin levels or irregularities in ovulation.

6.3 Factors affecting infertility

Fertility of a couple is defined as fertility of both the partners. High fertility of one partner, to some extent, can balance the low fertility in the other partner. Low fertility in both partners can however lead to first- or second-degree infertility [17].

Another significant factor influencing fertility is the age of the female partner. Fertility in both males and females is at its peak in the mid-twenties. In females, it starts to decline sharply after 30 years [2]. As many couples do not conceive a child at an early age, postponement of pregnancy decreases the number as well as the quality of egg, reducing the chances of getting pregnant. Females also go through an unwanted sequel of circumstances such as endometriosis, pelvic inflammatory disease (PID) and uterine fibrinoids. All these complications lead to the release of cytokines in the form of interleukins and C-reactive proteins, which further contribute to the already existing infertility in females [15].

It is not easy to determine the exact cause of infertility as there are many factors that bias. The cause can be recognised only after proper investigations.

6.4 Association of female infertility with hypothyroidism

Hypothyroidism is common in males and females. A range of reproductive disorders ranging from abnormal sexual growth to menstrual cycle irregularities or infertility have been connected to thyroid disorders. Morphological changes of follicles in hypothyroidism may be an outcome of higher prolactin production that blocks both secretion as well as action of gonadotropins [4]. Enough supplementation of thyroid hormone restores prolactin and normalises ovulatory function [3]. Hypothyroidism itself possibly will contribute to infertility because thyroid hormones may be necessary for maximum production of both oestradiol and progesterone hormones (**Figure 4**).

7. Obesity

Obesity represents excess body fat or is defined by a basal metabolic rate of more than 30 ky/m^2. Elevated levels of TSH; hypothyroidism does not always result in weight problems but may cause obesity in some cases.

Subclinical hypothyroidism, marked by elevated TSH concentration with normal concentration of peripheral thyroid hormones (T3 andT4) has been consistently found in obese individuals. Lipid profile findings of obese individuals show marked dyslipidemia, involving high levels of serum TG, LDL, TC and low serum HDL level [14]. A recent report from coronary artery risk development in young adults (CARDIA) shows that among physiologically infertile women, probability of infertility is twice in African and American women as compared to others [15]. Economic problems have led to limited access to diagnosis and treatment of various diseases, resulting in selective underestimation of thyroid dysfunctions and hypothyroidism related infertility [18].

Thyroid affects various aspects of reproduction; especially pregnancy is adversely affected by thyroid dysfunction [19].

An understanding of the implications of obesity and hormonal balance and fertility may help couples facing challenges in conception to give the reproductive health and better opportunity and take steps to improve the reproductive capacity and probability of a healthy pregnancy.

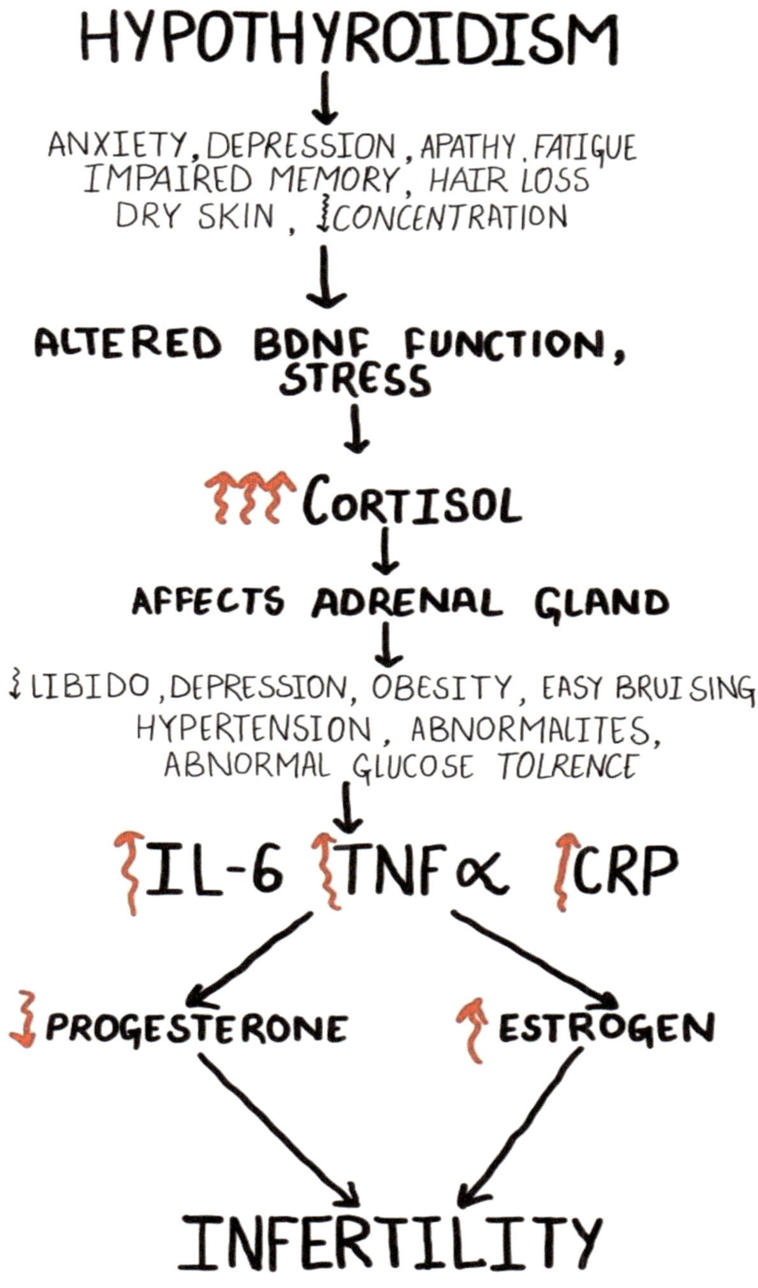

Figure 4.
Hypothyroidism and infertility. (Courtesy – Ms. Aparajita Kushwaha, Ms. Sanghapriya Mukherjee).

Consequences of obesity on ovarian function.

- Changed oestrogen metabolism.
- Insulin resistance.
- High androgen levels.

- Slim women are oestrogen deficient while obese women have an excess of oestrogen but have irregular cycles [20].
- BMI – more than 30 kg/m^2.
- Body fat affects the onset of puberty.

Obese adipocytes act as secretary cells and release adipose cytokines, chemokines and cytokines. The secretion of inflammatory agents like IL-6 and TNF-@ is considerably increased in obese individuals. These contribute towards producing a low-grade chronic systemic inflammation. Thyroid hormones can affect the metabolism of cholesterol and triglycerides, where depression of cholesterol concentrations caused due to an increase in hepatic LDL levels, or decreased LDL clearance can be seen. As a result, total cholesterol or LDL levels are increased in hypothyroid individuals.

Obesity is not only associated with infertility but also with various other health problems including hypertension, cardiovascular diseases, diabetes and hormonal imbalances. The effects of obesity expand across conception, gestation, parturition and also post-parturition. Excess weight gain negatively impacts efficacy of treatment and results of served reproductive techniques. Therefore, high body fat and obesity cause a rise in oestrogen production that body perceives as birth control confining the chances of acquiring pregnancy (**Figure** 5).

8. Stress

Stress is most common in women. Stress is normally underestimated because of dysfunction in reproduction. Stress-induced anovulation (SIA) usually termed

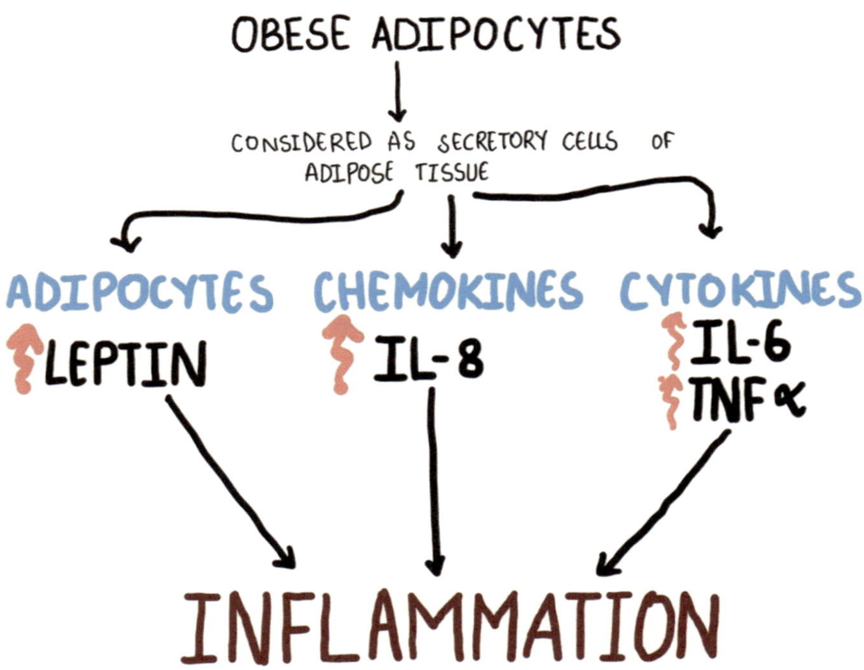

Figure 5.
Relationship between obesity and inflammation. (Courtesy – Ms. Aparajita Kushwaha, Ms. Sanghapriya Mukherjee).

functional hypothalamic amenorrhea (FHA) and functional chronic hypothalamic anovulation, which causes infertility, increases acute and chronic health burden in women of all ages.

Chronic psychological and physical stress is common among hypothyroid individuals. This causes an elevated production of cortisol which aggravates release of IL-6incirculation [21].

Increased level of IL-6 tends to suppress immune system and endocrine system. This is responsible for production of acute phase protein, i.e., CRP.

Effects of IL-6 are mediated through regression of BDNF (Brain-Derived Neurotropic Factor). Downregulation of BDNF causes decreased connectivity in between anterior singulating cortex and several limbic areas like hippocampus. Increased level of IL-6 in stress causes FHA (functional hypothalamic amenorrhea). This leads to defects in the mechanism operating the anterior pituitary gland resulting in delayed ovum maturation, decreased FSH and decreased LH, which results in infertility.

IL-6 synthesis through peripheral blood mononuclear cultures of chronically stressed individuals has been reported to be higher than that of cultures from control subjects when stimulated by LPS, in a study conducted on older adults [22].

IL6 is a multifunctional cytokine with essential roles in inflammatory response or in leading T-cell differentiation in acquired immunity. IL-6 is broadly expressed in reproductive tract or gestational tissues of women, as well as maintains a regulatory role in embryo implantation or placental development, and immune adaptations are required for tolerating pregnancy. Elevated IL-6 is recurrently evident in altered cytokine profiles, feature of unexplained infertility, recurrent miscarriage, preterm delivery and preeclampsia. Especially, there is undeniable evidence representing altered IL-6 trans-signalling in female prone to recurrent miscarriage, with higher IL-6 bioavailability potentially suppressing generation of CD4 cells and T-cells, regulatory cells necessary for tolerance of pregnancy.

Inadequate local IL-6 may also lead to fetal loss since IL-6 appearance is reduced in the endometrium of females due to recurrent miscarriage [23].

CRP is an acute phase response protein synthesised by liver. Small levels of CRP are present normally in blood but increase rapidly in response to inflammatory conditions [22]. Hypothyroidism can increase chronic subclinical inflammation which raises IL-6 levels, resulting in raised levels of CRP. Hypothyroidism is associated with relatively increased inflammatory marker levels [24]. Psychological stress causes a rise in CRP, which can lead to a poor prognosis as well as pregnancy complications [25].

Stress, eating habit and infertility:

Infertility often results in immense pressure leading to a lot of stress and anxiety. Depression tends to induce unhealthy eating habits. Due to excessive consumption of unhealthy food, it paves way to obesity and an increase in the level of the

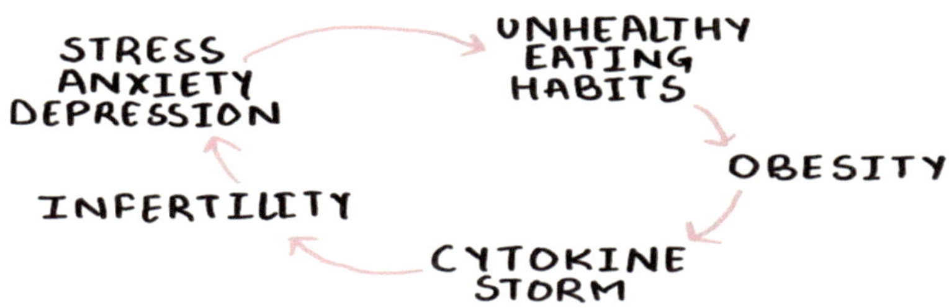
STRESS
ANXIETY
DEPRESSION
UNHEALTHY
EATING
HABITS
OBESITY
CYTOKINE
STORM
INFERTILITY

Figure 6.
Cytokine storm in hypothyroid subjects. Courtesy: Ms. Sanghapriya Mukherjee, Ms. Aparajita Kushwaha.

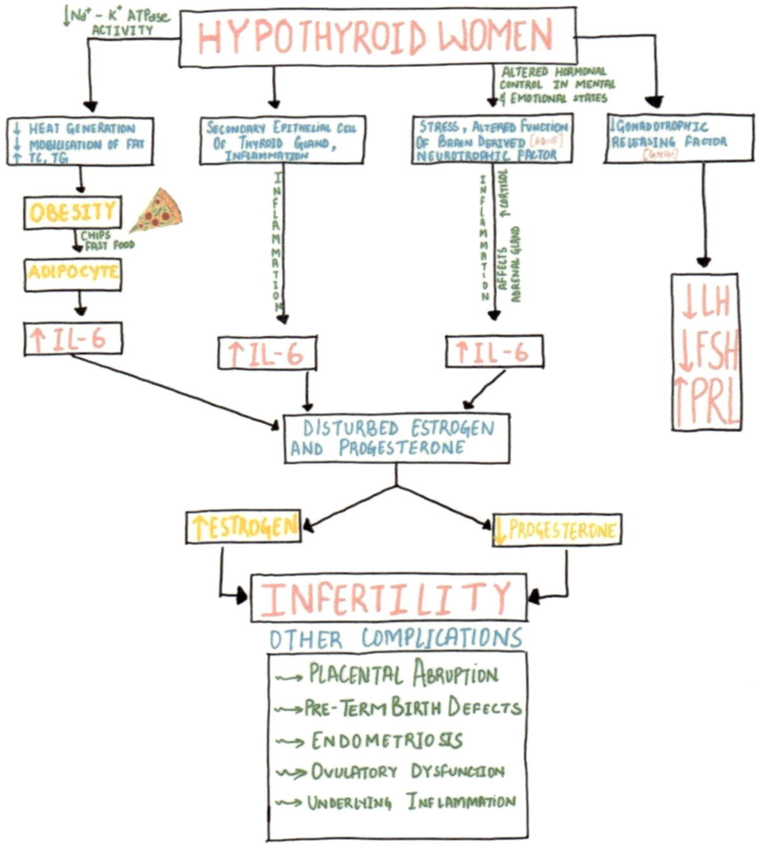

Figure 7.
Summary: hypothyroidism and infertility. (Picture courtesy: Dr. Neha Sharma).

inflammatory markers (cytokine storm), and finally resulting in probability of conception to almost zero (**Figures 6** and 7).

9. Conclusion

In women of reproductive age, hypothyroidism poses a great risk to their fertility. Hypothyroidism triggers a cascade of physiological irregularities and also makes women more prone to diseases.

Though obesity is not necessarily a part of symptoms and effect of hypothyroidism, it is not uncommon for hypothyroid women to be obese. Various factors contribute towards excess weight gain in hypothyroid women, mainly, hypothyroidism-induced depression and hormonal changes, which usually results in unhealthy eating habits and eventually weight gain. The accumulation of fat cells or obese adipocytes acts as secretary cells and secrete IL-8, IL-6 and TNF-α (inflammatory agents) causing a low-grade inflammatory response.

Hypothyroid women also suffer from chronic physiological and mental stress. Chronic stress causes elevated levels of cortisol which triggers increased secretion of inflammatory agents like IL-6 and CRP.

Hypothyroidism induces obesity, stress, anxiety and depression, thus cumulatively causes inflammation in the body, which leads to difficulty in conception, frequent miscarriages and infertility in severe cases.

Abbreviations

BDNF	Brain derived neurotropic factor
BMI	Body Mass Index
CARDIA	Coronary artery risk development in young adults
CD-4	Cluster of differentiation-4
CRP	C reactive protein
FHA	Functional hypothalamic amenorrhoea
FSH	Follicle stimulating hormone
GnRH	Gonadotropin releasing hormone
HDL	High density lipoprotein
IL-6	Interleukin-6
IVF	In vitro fertilisation
LH	Luteinizing hormone
LPS	Luteal phase ovarian stimulation
PCOD	Poly-cystic ovarian disease
PID	Pelvic inflammatory disease
SIA	Stress induced anovulation
TC	Total cholesterol
TG	Triglycerides
TNF	Tumour necrosis factor
TSH	Thyroid stimulating hormone
WHO	World Health Organisation

Author details

Neha Sharma*, Sanghapriya Mukherjee and Aparajita Kushwaha
Department of Biochemistry, Geetanjali Medical College and Hospital, Udaipur, Rajasthan, India

*Address all correspondence to: neha16.sharma@gmail.com

References

[1] Meyer BJ, Meiji H, Sand Meyer AC. Human Physiology. 2nd ed. Cape Town: Juta and Co, LTD; 1997

[2] Willocks J, Neilson JP. Obstetrics and Gynaecology. 4th ed. Edinburgh: Churchill Livingstone; 1997

[3] Carl AB, Edward RA, David EB, Tietz NW. Textbook of Clinical Chemistry and molecular diagnostics. 6th ed. Philadelphia: Elsevier Saunders Publishers; 2008. pp. 2021-2027

[4] Ferin M, Jewelewicz R, Warren M. The Menstrual Cycle: Physiology, Reproductive Disorder and Infertility. New York: Oxford University Press; 1993

[5] Crosignani PG, Colombo M, Vegetti W, Somiglinana E, Gressati A, Ragni G. Overweight and obese anovulatory patients with polycystic ovaries: Parallel improvements in anthropometric indices, ovarian physiology and fertility rate induced by diet. Human Reproduction. 2003;**18**:1928-1932

[6] Vannuccini S, Clifton VL, Fraser IS, Taylor HS, Critchley H, Giudice LC, Petraglia F. Infertility and reproductive disorders: Impact of hormonal and inflammatory mechanism on pregnancy outcome. Human Reproduction Update 2016;22(1):104-115

[7] Dhandapani K, Kodavanji B, Vinodini NA. Association of Body Mass Index with primary and secondary infertility among infertile women in Mangalore: A cross-sectional study. National Journal of Physiology, Pharmacy and Pharmacology. 2016; **6**(1):81-84

[8] De Groot LJ, Jameson JL. Endocrinology. 4th ed. Vol. 3. Philadelphia, PA: Elsevier/Saunders; 2005

[9] De Groot LJ, Jameson JL. Low density lipoprotein and risk of myocardial infarction circulation. Endocrinology. 1997;**96**:2520-2515

[10] Chen G, Lin Y, Huang B, Yao J, Jiang Q, Wen J, et al. Association between cardiovascular risk, insulin resistance, b-cell function and thyroid dysfunction: A cross-sectional studyin the she ethnic minority group of Fujian province in China. European Journal of Endocrinology. 2010;**163**:775-782

[11] Amela B, Edina BK. The importance of Hba1c control in patients with sub-clinical hypothyroidism. Materia Socio-Medica. 2012;**24**(4):212-219

[12] Hollowell JG, Staehling NW, Flanders WD. Serum TSH, T4 and thyroid antibodies in the United States population (1988 to 1994) National Health and Nutrition Examination Survey (NHANES). Journal of Clinical Endocrinology and Metabolism 2002, 87 (@):489-499

[13] Lauren PR, Terry FD. Hypothyroidism and Thyroiditis. Williams Text Book of Endocrinology. 10th ed. Philadelphia: WB Saunders; 2002. pp. 423-448

[14] Brugh VM, Nudell DM, Lipschultz LI. What the urologist should know about the female infertility evaluation. Urologic Clinics of North America. 2002;**29**(4):983-992

[15] Tindall VR. Jeffcoate's Principles of Gynaecology. 5th ed. London: Butterworths; 1987

[16] Pearce EN, Andersson M, Zimmermann MB. Global iodine nutrition: Where do we stand in 2013? Thyroid. 2013;**23**(5):523-528

[17] Franz MJ, Bantle JP, Beebe CA, Brunzell JD, Chiasson JL, Garg A, et al. Evidence based nutrition principles and

recommendations for the treatment and prevention of diabetes and related complications. Diabetes Care. 2002;**25**: 148-198

[18] Wischmann TH. Psychogenic infertility-Myths and facts. Journal of Assisted Reproduction and Genetics. 2003;**20**(12):484-494

[19] Martinez GM, Chandra A, Amba JC, Jones J, Mosher WD. Fertility, contraception and fatherhood: Data on men and women from cycle 6. National Survey of Family Growth. Vital and Health Statistics. 2006;**23**(26):1-142

[20] Krassas GE, Pontikides N, Kaltsas T, Papadopoulou P, Paunkovic J, Paunkovic N. Disturbances of menstruation in hypothyroidism. Clinical Endocrinology. 1999;**50**(5): 655-659

[21] Wang JX, Davies M, Norman RJ. Body mass and probability of pregnancy during assisted reproductive treatment. British Medical Journal. 2000;**10**:551-554

[22] Banks WA, Kastin AJ, Gutierrze EG. Penetration of interleukin-6 across the murine blood brain barrier. Neuroscience Letters. 1994;**179**(1–2): 53-56

[23] Miller GE, Cohen S, Ritchey AK. Chronic psychological stress and the regulation of pro-inflammatory cytokines: A glucocorticoid-resistance model. Health Psychology. 2002;**21**(6): 531-541

[24] Christ-Crain M, Meier C, Guglielmetti M, Huber PR, Riesen W, Staub JJ, et al. Elevated C-reactive protein and homocysteine values: Cardioavscular risk factorsin hypothyroidism? A cross-sectional and a double blinded, placebo-controlled trial. Atherosclerosis. 2003;**166**(2):379-386

[25] Coussans-Read ME, Okum ML, Nettles CD. Psychological stress increase inflammation markers and alters cytokine production across pregnancy. Brain, Behavior, and Immunity. 2007; **21**:343-350

Chapter 8

Evolution of Thyroid Enhancement of Embryogenesis and Early Survival

Arjay Pataueg, Earl T. Larson and Christopher L. Brown

Abstract

Iodine imparts protective antioxidant actions that improve the fitness of invertebrate organisms, and peptides carrying iodine initially appear to have served in a defensive capacity. Tyrosine carries multiple iodines in some echinoderms, and these peptides transferred to progeny serve both protective and signaling purposes. This parental relationship appears to be the most likely evolutionary basis for emergence of the vertebrate thyroid endocrine system, and its critically important development-promoting actions in larval and (later) fetal ontogeny. Thyroxine (T_4) and Triiodothyronine (T_3) induce settlement and stimulate transitions to alternative feeding modes in some echinoderms. This transgenerational relationship has been conserved and elaborated in vertebrates, including humans, which share common ancestry with echinoderms. Thyroid insufficiency is damaging or can be lethal to larval fishes; egg yolk that is insufficiently primed with maternal thyroid hormones (TH) results in compromised development and high mortality rates at the time of first-feeding. Maternally-derived TH supplied to offspring supports the onset of independent feeding in fishes (eye, mouth, lateral line, swim bladder and intestinal maturation) and survival by comparable developmental mechanisms in placental mammals. Fishes evolved precise control of TH secretion and peripheral processing; early metamorphic and feeding mode actions were joined by controlled thermogenesis in homeotherms.

Keywords: Thyroid hormone, T_3, T_4, embryogenesis, larvae, fetus, metamorphosis, survival

1. Introduction

Thyroid hormones have historically been associated with their thermoregulatory roles [1] and with the control of metamorphosis, as classically described in frogs [2]. A critically important role in human fetal development [3] is also well known, and is the basis for extensive thyroid status testing of pregnant women, and for the widespread use of iodized salt [4]. Comparative and evolutionary perspectives on thyroid regulatory biology had a relatively recent arrival. The ability to measure thyroid hormones [5] led to analysis of patterns of regulatory involvement not only in amphibian metamorphoses and human fetal development, but far more broadly among vertebrates throughout early differentiation. The origin of these actions seen throughout the vertebrates can be traced to consistent associations of thyroid hormones with the successful transition from larval to juvenile forms, generally accompanied by transitions to different modes of feeding and nutrition, or movement to different habitats. Recent research suggests that larval stimulation and signaling by iodinated peptides originated in invertebrates, and that the substantial survival implications of this form of maternal chemical communication in offspring ensured its evolutionary retention [6]. Conversely, it follows that the untoward consequences of hypothyroidism can be severe or lethal. The harsh impacts of hypothyroidism in fetal humans originated in connections between iodinated peptide signaling and successful larval differentiation in advanced invertebrates, a trait that has been consistently conserved and elaborated among the vertebrata. Insufficient human maternal thyroid stimulation results in the tragic syndrome known as cretinism [3], characterized by extremely deficient fetal development, central nervous system disorders, severe retardation, abnormal digestive and skeletal differentiation, stunting, lethargy, and a sharply reduced lifespan.

2. Evolutionary origins of the vertebrate thyroid system

Iodide is a large and biologically active anion, with a capacity to reduce reactive oxygen species, and it performs protective antioxidant functions in a range of invertebrate and algal organisms [7]. It is also involved in numerous biosynthetic activities. Some multicellular organisms concentrate iodide and it is often found bound to proteins or peptides [8], particularly the amino acid tyrosine, which can carry multiple iodides. Tyrosine is derived from phenylalanine and can be processed further into dopamine and other catecholamines, and it is essential for the synthesis of thyroid hormones tri-iodothyronine (T_3) and thyroxin (T_4). The latter two compounds consist of paired tyrosine residues with three or four attached iodides, respectively.

Tyrosines become iodinated spontaneously in marine environments, and are found throughout marine invertebrates. T_4 synthesis is an ancient process, occurring when iodinated tyrosines are coupled together, and some invertebrate physiological functions have been tentatively ascribed to it [9]. Iodinated signaling is an antiquated process, probably beginning with receptors in invertebrates responding to exogenous iodinated tyrosines coming from either seawater or marine algae [10]. Certain mollusks have been found to possess genes for peroxidases, one of which is similar to thyroid peroxidase, which binds iodine to thyroglobulin in vertebrates. While mollusks do not have thyroglobulin, one of their peroxidases incorporates iodine into thyroid hormone-like molecules. This may reflect the first incidence of endogenous production of thyroid like-hormones [11]. Specialized cells for the processing of iodinanted tyrosines are present in protochordates, and are organized into thyroid-like tissues, e.g. the endostyle [12]. In agnathans, the larval endostyle is retained and reorganized in adult lampreys into thyroid follicles with iodine-concentrating capacity. Lamprey metamorphosis is at least partly thyroid hormone-driven, and is characterized by a transition from larval filter feeding to ingestion of captured materials, and the larval endostyle is altered after metamorphosis into a thyroid gland with functional follicles [13]. Interestingly, the endostyle in lampreys develops around the time of yolk sac absorption [14]. In the other cyclostome group, hagfish, the thyroid primordium appears in the area of the head adjacent to the yolk sac [15]. These examples suggest a possibility of maternal thyroid signaling in larval cyclostomes.

An emerging body of evidence suggests that signaling by iodinated tyrosines was linked to changes in feeding modes before the evolution of protochordates and chordates, and that numerous physiological functions of thyroid- and thyroid-like iodinated peptides can be found in echinoderms. Maternal / larval signaling in the echinoderms may be the ancestral origin of the maternal / juvenile regulatory relationship that prevails throughout the vertebrates, and which figures prominently in *Homo sapiens*.

2.1 Echinoderms: Iodothyronines in larval signaling

Although echinoderms have relatively simple anatomical characteristics, their embryos are classified as deuterostomes, which means the mouth develops after the anus, and chordates are also classified thusly [6]. For this reason, they are thought to share a common ancestry with chordates [16]. This common ancestor has not yet been identified but some ideas of its characteristics are being deduced using comparative genomics [17]. Iodinated tyrosines, including thyroxin, are found in a variety of living tissues including monocellular algae [18] and echinoderm embryos [19], where there is ample evidence of maternal signals carrying out beneficial regulatory roles in early development [20, 21]. A good case can be made for the echinoderms having evolved a regulatory mechanism in development that enabled progeny to respond to signals by shifting developmental modes and feeding patterns, a pattern of transgenerational communication which has been conserved to contribute later to the adaptation of juvenile vertebrates to diverse and changing environments [22].

Some evidence supports the hypothesis that dietary sources of iodide served initially as antioxidants and evolutionarily later as signaling mechanisms to promote DNA expression, thereby initiating and facilitating successful invertebrate metamorphoses [6]. Because these actions promote changes that distinctly enhance the rate of larval survival, their selective value is high and these traits promote their own conservation and propagation. Most echinoderms distribute free-swimming larvae that mature, metamorphose, and settle as benthic organisms; some are dependent on exogenous feeding prior to settlement, while others can metamorphose without feeding [20]. Many echinoderm larvae exhibit changes in developmental rate or status and distinct modifications of their developmental mode in response to iodothyronines including exogenous thyroid hormones. Exogenous T_3 and T_4 both accelerate development, metamorphosis and settlement in sand dollars (*Leodia sexiesperforata*), and appear to facilitate a transition from obligate larval feeding to an alternative mode in which metamorphosis occurs independently of exogenous nutrition [21], foretelling important advancements in vertebrate reproduction. The capacity for endogenous TH synthesis is theorized to have replaced dependence on dietary TH (an exogenous messenger), facilitating the endocrine regulation of larval development, and generating some degree of internal control over the induction of metamorphosis [19]. Endogenous synthesis of TH has been confirmed in larval sand dollars (*L. sexiesperforata*), sea biscuits (*Clypeaster rosaceus*), and sea urchins (*Strongylocentrotus purpuratus*) [21].

The role of iodinated tyrosine shifts in echinoderms from the provision of iodine for protective purposes and responsiveness to exogenous signals, to the emergence of a regulatory endocrine system that can alter the timing of physiological and morphological changes to increase developmental competence. In the case of sea urchins, exposure to either exogenous or endogenous T_4 promotes the initiation of larval exoskeleton synthesis [21].

The effectiveness of larval regulatory signaling by TH is dependent not only on the availability of hormones of either exogenous (dietary or maternal iodotyrosines) or endogenous origin (TH biosynthesis). In the case of sea urchins, activation of the MAPK protein kinase pathway occurs after binding of thyroxin to receptors [21]. Genes for hormone receptors, appropriate intracellular response mechanisms, deiodinase enzymes and other components may be required. The roles of these signals in the acquisition of metamorphic capability in relation to exogenous larval feeding [11] is the fundamental relationship that has been conserved throughout evolution for the promotion of GI system and other physiological adaptations, enabling successful transition to exogenous feeding in fishes [22, 23] and higher vertebrates. The ancestral deuterostome likely laid the foundation for regulation of the timing of larval metamorphoses in teleost fishes, as closely associated with the initiation of exogenous feeding. We see this pattern conserved in both echinoderms [24, 25] and hemichordates [26]. These groups comprise ambulacraria, the sister clade of chordates [27].

2.2 Hemichordates: Iodine or bromine?

Hemichordates (acorn worms) are the sister group to echinoderms in the ambulacraria, the sister clade of chordates. Hemichordates and echinoderms diverged approximately 876 mya whereas ambulacraria diverged from chordates 896 mya [27]. While one species of acorn worm (not actual worms), *Saccoglossus horsti*, has been shown to iodinate tyrosine by incorporating I^{131} into monoiodotyrosine [28], other species seem to manage this process differently. Acorn worms of the genera *Ptychodera*, *Glossobalanus* and *Balanoglossus*, use bromine instead of iodine [29]. They brominate indoles and phenols, the bromoindoles being similar to iodoindoles in other species. These halogenated phenols give the animals a characteristic smell described by many as iodophoric [29]. These chemicals seem to serve an antiseptic role rather than any sort of metabolic or metamorphic role [29]. Instead, embryogenesis and metamorphosis in indirect developing acorn worms seems to be controlled by FGF (firbroblast growth factor) [30]. Therefore, if iodothyronine control is a basal deuterostome trait, then it seems to be lost in hemichordates. An alternate explanation is that it was evolved separately in echinoderms and chordates. Much more work needs to be done on this group to elucidate whether other species consolidate iodine and if actors other than FGF play a role in embryogenesis and metamorphosis.

2.3 Protochordates: TRIAC and an endostyle

Protochordates are one of the three members of the phylum chordata along with urochordates (tunicates) and vertebrates. They are considered to be the basal chordate group [31]. The representative member of this group is the lancelet (Amphioxus), comprised by two genera, *Branchiostoma* and *Asymmetron.* The active form of iodinated tyrosine in amphioxus is triiodothryoacetic acid (TRIAC), rather than the triiodothyronine (T_3) used among vertebrates [12]. TRIAC differs from T_3 by having only two rings instead of three. Both T_4 and T_3 are found in amphioxous, but it is TRIAC, a metabolite of T_3 that is the active form [32]. T_4 is converted peripherally to T_3 by deiodination and T_3 is converted to TRIAC by deamination [33]. Amphioxus embryos lack large amounts of yolk and extra-embryonic tissues. This sets them apart from the vertebrates and is thought to be a basal chordate trait [31]. As far as the authors know, no studies have been done on thyroid hormone content of protochordate yolk. It is entirely possible that TH could be present in the yolk and it has not been detected as of yet. It is important to note that in ambulacraria, direct developing larvae have large amounts of yolk and indirect developing (planktonic) larvae do not [32, 34].

It is established that TRIAC controls the metamorphosis of amphioxus from a pelagic larva to a benthic post-larva [35, 36]. Metamorphosis is triggered by TRIAC binding to thyroid hormone receptors (TR). The expression of these receptors is greatest just before metamorphosis [33]. In amphioxous, the endostyle is the site of T_4 production. The endostyle has already been thought to be the thyroid homolog in larval cyclostomes [13], but the endostyle appears to be serving as a thyroid homolog in both larval and adult amphioxous [12]. As previously stated, T_4 and T_3 are produced in the endostyle and metabolized in the periphery. To be more specific, this deiodination and deamination takes place in the hepatic caecum, which is thought to be the homolog of the vertebrate liver [12]. Indeed, in vertebrates T_4 is converted to T_3 in the liver [8].

2.4 Maternal thyroid signaling in larval fishes

Female fishes deposit thyroid hormones against a concentration gradient in eggs during ovarian maturation [37]. Larval fishes are completely dependent on thyroid hormones of maternal origin until endogenous biosynthesis begins, and the regulatory capacity of the thyroid system has been attained. From that point forward, the thyroid system products in juvenile fishes have roles in organ system maturation, and the functionality of that system becomes dependent on adequate dietary sources of iodine [23].

Groupers are a family of marine fishes with small larvae that require relatively small food organisms. Cultured larval groupers are subject to large-scale mortality at the time of first feeding, but a switch from cultured rotifers to wild copepods provides a much more substantial supply of iodine, in response to which a sharp increase in larval survival has been attributed [38]. Some investigators have ascribed initial successes with larval groupers using copepods as a first feed entirely to differences in nutritional content [39], although iodine content of copepods and enhancement of digestive enzyme secretion in response to the copepod diet have been noted by other investigators [40]. These end-points are entirely consistent with established endocrine regulatory responses to micronutrient deficiencies in captive-reared populations, as reviewed previously [41] and as discussed further, below.

Thyroid hormones stimulate an integrated complex of developmental events that are crucial for early survival, collectively enabling fish larvae to make the transition from yolk absorption to active feeding [23]. Sensory, locomotor and digestive system maturation are essential for active feeding, and mortality on a substantial scale routinely occurs in captivity around the time of initial feeding [40]. In some cases, that has been attributed to an insufficiency of maternally-derived thyroid hormones [42, 43], sometimes in response to dietary iodine deficiencies. Perception of food items depends in part on eye and lateral line function, and olfactory organ input; pursuit of prey involves efficient swimming and neutral buoyancy, and the processing of food, absorption and utilization of nutrients hinge on the effective production of digestive enzymes. The maturation of the aforementioned physiological systems is strongly regulated by thyroid hormones of maternal origin, and all of these mechanisms become active on or slightly before the time of first-feeding [44, 45]. Early maturational events in the central nervous system are also dependent on maternally-derived thyroid hormones, enabling the processing of and responsiveness to critically important information.

2.5 Functional sensory systems

The detection of potential prey items by larvae typically involves mechanosensory detection of vibrations by the lateral line and the use of vision and/or smell to locate potential prey. The thyroid axis promotes neuromast proliferation and maturation and induces expansion of the neuromast population in the trunk in zebrafish [46]. First-feeding typically occurs around day 5 in zebrafish, and is coincident with the onset of visual, lateral line, and locomotor function and acquisition of the capacity to digest prey organisms. The onset of lateral line function requires maturation of neuromasts, as well as peripheral nerve transmission and processing by the central nervous system (CNS). In addition to the development of lateral line components, maternally-derived thyroid hormones promote differentiation and maturational changes in the CNS [47, 48].

The eyes also differentiate and become functional in response to maternal thyroid signaling, just before the onset of feeding in zebrafish [45]. Experimental applications of Insulin-like Growth Factor-1 (IGF-1) receptor blockers and analysis of IGF-1 gene expression revealed that eye differentiation in response to maternal TH signaling is transduced by IGF-1. Treatment with exogenous TH causes expression of IGF-1 genes, thereby accelerating initial eye function by up to three or four days [45]. A parallel assortment of somatosensory deficiencies is reported in response to mammalian neonatal hypothyroidism [46].

2.6 Locomotor system maturation

Fin maturation is characterized by the development of fin rays and changes in the morphology of dorsal, caudal and other fins beginning just after hatching, as embyronic forms proceed in transitions into free-swimming larvae [49]. Fins and scales are established targets for thyroid-induced maturation [50, 51] and their functionality is critically important in the successful transition to autonomous feeding. Skeletal development in fins is homologous with vertebrate limb bone development [52], and regulatory actions appear to be homologous. Hypothyroid mammals are subject to severely compromised locomotor function, with evidence of musculoskeletal deficiencies, exaggerated behavioral and cognitive inhibition, and displays of increased immobility and anxiety-related behaviors [53].

In addition to fin and musculoskeletal development, buoyancy is essential for energy-efficient pursuit of prey. Larval fishes with undifferentiated or uninflated swim bladders are unable to swim efficiently and they can readily become a component of the heavy mortalities associated with failed transitions to first feeding. Swim bladder ontogeny and inflation are under the control of maternal thyroid hormones [42, 43], and TH-induced swimbladder maturation and initial function are transduced by IGF-1, as is eye development [45]. A significant improvement in swimbladder inflation rate is attributed to TH exposure [42] and a strong relationship ($p < 0.005$) was reported between egg T_3 content and survival to two weeks post-hatching in striped bass (*Morone saxatilis*), with a correlation coefficient of 0.922 [42]. Mammalian lungs are evolutionary derivatives of the piscene swim bladder, and functional use of modified swim bladders for respiratory purposes is widespread among taxonomically diverse fishes [52]. Respiratory failures are listed among responses to hypothyroidism in humans, which according to the American Thyroid Association can result in lung function slowing "to the point that they can no longer keep up critical function" [54].

2.7 Production of digestive enzymes

Aquisition of the capability to find and ingest food does not ensure larval survival; numerous cases have been reported of larvae ingesting zooplankton or other organisms followed by failures to process, absorb and utilize their nutritional content. Maturation of the intestine is also controlled by maternal thyroid signals, and in cases in which those signals are lost or weakened, acutely underdeveloped and frail larvae with poor prospects for survival can be produced. In the Japanese eel *Anguilla japonica*, for example, Kurokawa et al. [55] observed that eel leptocephali started feeding at day 7 and reportedly found ingested rotifers in larvae up to 13 days of age with no physical or immunohistochemical evidence of digestion or absorption. Growth in these leptocephali essentially stops at the completion of yolk absorption on day 7, and is usually followed by mortality within a few days [55]. Larval Anguillids are notoriously difficult to rear in captivity, and practical closure of the eel life cycle has eluded hatchery technologists for more than half a century. One possible explanation is that adult eels that mature in captivity fail to deposit adequate stimulatory endocrine signals into their eggs [56], producing seriously hypothyroid larvae with debilitating developmental deficiencies, including a sharply reduced capacity to produce digestive enzymes.

Increasing the content of the thyroid hormone T_3 in marine fish eggs advanced the timing of the onset of digestive function, and significantly improved the rate of survival [57]. Further study of numerous species of larval fishes revealed that the expression of genes encoding digestive enzymes was induced by thyroid hormones [58, 59] coincident with the time of first feeding, which was interpreted as an indication that maternal signaling is a critically important determinant of the onset of intestinal digestive competence and consequently of survival. It is noteworthy that extensive and debilitating digestive system deficiencies and often acute failures are routinely reported in humans in response to hypothyroidism [60].

2.8 Maternal endocrine status is a prime determinant of egg quality

Egg quality was a characteristic of fish eggs that for many years had a circular definition – egg quality was defined as the capability of eggs to produce viable larvae for reasons that were speculatively considered and often dismissed as technically out of reach. Poor egg quality was attributed in earlier reviews to a combination of unknown genetic and nutritional variables, but regulatory materials such as endocrine signaling compounds (hormones and maternal mRNAs) were not yet being considered [61]. Thyroid signals deposited in fish eggs were recognized by some investigators as key determinants of egg quality more than 25 years ago [44] although numerous recent analyses of egg quality have completely overlooked the contribution of maternal thyroid hormones to larval success.

Some fish species are very reluctant to spawn in captivity, and captive-reared fishes released into wild environments often exhibit substantially compromised reproductive performance [62]. An inhibitory dopanimergic neural pathway is activated in response to a variety of stresses including environmental alterations, resulting in blockage of gonadotropin synthesis and release and imparied reproductive competence [63]. The degree of inhibition is variable, ranging from no inhibition whatsoever to erratic reproductive performance to complete reproductive failure. For this reason, challenging species are often treated with Ovaprim, the innovative spawning inducer developed by R. Peter and H-R Lin, which combines GnRH analogs and a dopamine receptor blocker [64]. Nevertheless, fertile eggs that produce larvae capable of hatching are not necessarily adequately provisioned with essential regulatory compounds to negotiate larval-juvenile metamorphoses. For these reasons, additional attention should be paid to the adequacy of maternal endocrine status during oogenesis.

Some species such as the striped bass (*M. saxatilis*) display highly variable production of viable eggs in captivity; two nearly identical-looking gravid females can display fertility rates of 4% and 94% (personal observation, unpublished). This may reflect variable endocrine status of broodstock females, since the deposition of essential regulatory hormones during oogenesis is determined by patterns of circulating hormones in maternal fishes. Larval survival in this species is highly dependent on the concentration of T_3 maternally deposited into eggs [42, 43]. Maternal endocrine status during ovarian maturation can be severely altered by variations in dietary iodine, stress, and other factors. For example, the iodine content of wild marine zooplankton was vastly higher than that of conventional aquaculture feeds, and a 700-fold concentration difference was reported in a comparison with *Artemia*. This difference was reflected in reduced circulating TH levels and an increased frequency of developmental deformities in *Artemia*-fed larval Atlantic halibuts (*Hippoglossus hippoglossus*) [65].

2.9 The net effect of maternally-stimulated sensory, locomotor, and digestive developments

The combined effect of maternally-derived thyroid stimulation during yolk absorption is the maturation of sensory (mechanoreceptor and visual) organs, fins and the swimbladder, and advancement of the timing of the onset of digestive capacity. These maturational events, together with maturation of CNS processing capability, convey a sharply increased degree of larval fitness and a much more likely successful transition to independent feeding.

Nearly complete mortality has been reported for some larval marine teleost cohorts, under both wild and hatchery conditions. In some cases, wild larvae reportedly have nearly no chance of survival during the yolk absorptive and early feeding phases, even in the absence of predators [66]. Early failure of large cohorts profoundly impacts recruitment strength and can shift patterns of speciation. Attention to and management of maternal thyroid provisioning of fish eggs has reportedly increased larval survival by up to five-fold [42].

The survival value imparted by endocrine regulatory contact with mother fishes has probably been a driving factor in the emergence of viviparity, which has occurred repeatedly among phylogenetically diverse fishes [23]. Prolonging the exposure of offspring to maternal hormones can result in nearly complete survival among the relatively mature K-selected progeny of live-bearing fishes. More primitive shark species are oviparous, but in the relatively modern viviparous placental sharks, maternal thyroid hormones are transferred to developing larvae over longer periods of time, where they promote advancements of growth, maturation, and development of juveniles [67].

Rudimentary signaling is done in echinoderms with iodinated tyrosine, in some cases with double-stranded thryoxin molecules. Protochordates show a leap forward with an actual organ, the endostyle, and production of T_4, T_3, peripheral deiodination and deamination and TRIAC signaling. However, neither of these are subject to the fine regulation found in vertebrate thyroid systems. Fishes evolved numerous thyroid-related mechanisms that are characteristic of sophisticated vertebrate endocrine systems, including efficient hormone synthesis with thryoglobulin (T_G), pituitary control of TH synthesis, hypothalamic control of pituitary regulatory mechanisms, sensitive multi-level feedback adjustment to regulate hormone synthesis and secretion, binding proteins, multiple hormone receptors, and an elaborate system of regulatory devices involved in the peripherial processing of TH. These can alter the ratios of highly biologically active T_3 to the much less potent T_4, as one means of fine-tuning local hormone concentrations and resultant levels of hormone activity. Most T_3 is derived from the deiodination of T_4, and monodeiodination can generate the much more highly biologically active T_3. It is also possible to deiodinate T_4 into the biologically inactive isomer reverse-T_3 (rT_3), as reported in some teleosts [68]. For these reasons T_4 has become recognized as essentially a prohormone that is capable of being processed into alternative endocrine products [69] with variable degrees of bioactivity. One net effect is that changing T_3/T_4 ratios can be precisely regulated as needed, and these ratios serve in higher vertebrates as indicative of metabolic states and thyroid system health.

Regulation of larval differentiation providing competence for first feeding is subject to some degree of plasticity. Glucocorticoids have some capacity to alter thyroid system activity by influencing the deiodination mechanisms mentioned above, thereby increasing the magnitude of generation of T_3. It has been proposed that alterations in maternally-circulating cortisol and other glucocorticoids can modify thyroid system function in ways that have adaptive value to fish embryos and larvae [70], by accelerating or delaying larval metamorphoses. Small alterations in the rate or timing of development can result in disproportionately large changes in anatomical or physiological outcomes, contributing importantly to adaptive radiation [52]. Integration of patterns of change in circulating thyroid and corticoid hormones have been reported in amphibian and flatfish metamorphoses, and the two endocrine systems are suspected to be functionally integrated [71].

An endocrine system with such precise control mechanisms emerged in fishes with a vital protective role toward offspring, and has been conserved. The finely-tuned control of thyroid bioactivity described above was adapted in a straightforward manner to the roles TH play in thermogenesis among birds and mammals [72].

Among important cellular mechanisms of action of maternal TH signals, many are mediated by hormonal stimulation of mitochondria. We have reported both the proliferation and activation of mitochondria in larvae in response to maternal TH signals, particularly in the intestine, the swimbladder, and neuromast cells of the lateral line [72]. Mitochondrial stimulation appears to be the basis for controlled thermogenesis in mammals, in specially-adapted brown fat tissues that evolved. It therefore appears likely that the elaboration of thyroid function initially for the enhancement of larval survival at the time of first feeding provided the mechanistic and regulatory basis needed for the later genesis of precisely-controlled thermogenesis.

3. Evolutionary implications of maternal thyroid contributions

Maternal/larval regulatory signaling has been described with an emphasis on the emergence of such interactions in advanced invertebrates, protochordates and lower vertebrates. This relationship has profound survival implications and has been retained and amplified in higher vertebrates, including humans. Comparative views of the origin and prototypical functions of physiological and biochemical interactions during development are briefly summarized in **Table 1**; a comparative perspective can be of substantial practical value [52].

Among reproducing fishes, a suite of adaptive developmental changes profoundly alters the likelihood of a successful transition from yolk absorption to exogenous feeding. Survival of this process is most likely if sensory, swimming, and digestive physiology are activated simultaneously prior to or at the time of first feeding. Visual and lateral line sensitivity, functional fins, a fully-inflated swim bladder, and the maturation of digestive enzyme secretory capability all contribute to the acquisition of nutrients after the exhaustion of yolk supplies. The development and early maturation of all of these physiological systems is under the control of thyroid signals of maternal origin that are deposited in yolk. Deficiencies of maternally-derived TH can have lethal consequences, especially in the transition to first-feeding. None of these peripheral or mechanistic functionalities are of value without effectient central processing, and regulation of the early maturation of the CNS is a major role of maternal endocrine regulation.

Taxonomic group		
Some echinoderms	**Fishes**	**Mammalia (humans)**
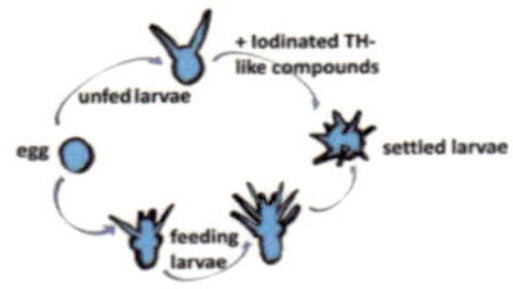	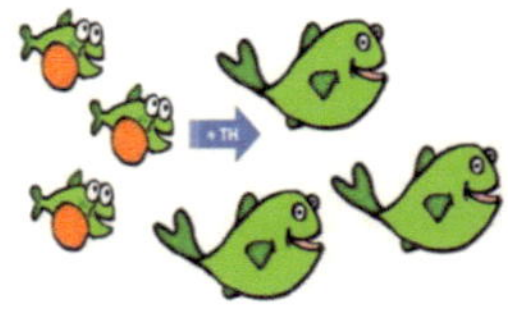	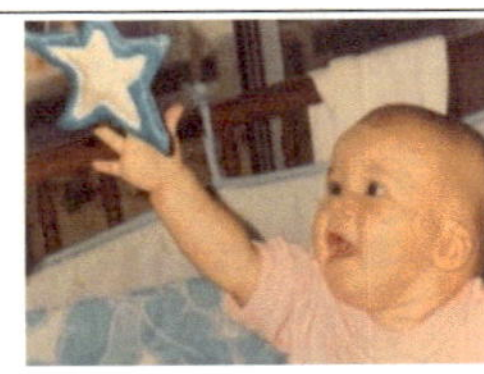
Outcomes		
↑ Metamorphosis, settlement independent of larval feeding	↑ survival of larval metamorphosis	↑ early growth, robust neuromuscular health
Maternally-derived chemical messengers		
TH-like iodinated peptides	Thyroid Hormones, cortisol	Thyroid Hormones, cortisol
Adaptive advantages, survival implications		
induction of metamorphosis control of settlement control, onset of feeding	CNS maturation sensory, motor integration	CNS maturation cognitive ability
New hormone targets, maturational processes		
metamorphic regulatory genes	swim bladder inflation digestive enzyme synthesis nutrient absorption lateral line function eye maturation mouth and teeth differentiation fins & locomotor mechanisms	respiratory function neural, physical integrity vigorous development sensory integration
Mechanisms evolved		
control of larval settlement	regulation of metamorphosis thyroid follicles pituitary hypothalamic control TH system feedback peripheral processing	thermoregulation

Table 1.
Evolutionary advancement of maternal regulation of larval/fetal ontogeny.

Maternal hormonal regulation of the fitness of offspring is so directly relevant to survival that it has been retained and amplified throughout vertebrate evolution. Specific consequences of neonatal hypothyroidism are numerous and can collectively be lethal, whether considered in the context of larval fishes or human infants. Central nervous system differentiation, the maturation of sensory, digestive, and locomotor organ systems all respond to maternal signaling, and they collectively facilitate transitions from embryonic and larval existence to more autonomous juvenile life.

4. Conclusions

Antioxidant functions of iodine generated a set of benefits to the parental transfer of iodinated compounds to offspring, eventually giving rise to the use of iodinated tyrosines for this purpose. These iodinated amino acids, in some cases in the form known in vertebrates as thyroid hormones, assumed signaling roles in some echinoderms, triggering metamorphic changes and alterations of modes of feeding. These signal-driven changes had substantial phenotypic value with advantages to survival, and consequently have been observed multiple times in echinoderms and chordates. Maternal provisioning of fish eggs provides a means of promoting development, altering the timing of metamorphosis and enhancing survival at the time of first-feeding, with some degree of plasticity. Regulatory maternal endocrine relationships with offspring have been retained in humans and other vertebrates, in which they are essential for normal development and survival.

Acknowledgements

Stipends in support of the investigators were provided by FAO World Fisheries University (WFU) Pilot Programme, and are deeply appreciated. Facilities and some supplies were made available by the WFU Pilot Programme, for which we are grateful. Professor Charles Bai generously shared research facilities with us, enabling our spawning and rearing of larval zebrafish to proceed.

Conflict of interest

The authors declare no conflict of interest.

Author details

Arjay Pataueg[1†], Earl T. Larson[2†] and Christopher L. Brown[1*]

1 FAO World Fisheries Programme, Pukyong National University, Busan, South Korea

2 Department of Biological Sciences, St. Johns River State College, Orange Park, Florida, USA

*Address all correspondence to: brownchristopher38@gmail.com

† These authors contributed equally to this work.

References

[1] Toni R. Ancient views on the hypothalamic–pituitary-thyroid axis: an historical and epistemological perspective. 2000;Pituitary 3(2):83-95. doi: 10.1023/a:1009953723963.

[2] Gudernatsch JF. Feeding experiments on tadpoles. I. The influence of specific organs given as food on growth and differentiation. A contribution to the knowledge of organs with internal secretion. 1912;Ach. Entwicklungsmech., Org., 35: 457-481.

[3] Patel J, Landers K, Li H, Mortimer RH and Richard K. Thyroid hormones and fetal neurological development. 2011;Journal of Endocrinology 209: 1-8.

[4] Moleti M, Lo Presti VP, Campolo MC, Mattina F, Galletti M, Mandolfino M, Violi MA, Giorgianni G, De Domenico D, Trimarchi F, Vermiglio F. Iodine prophylaxis using iodized salt and risk of maternal thyroid failure in conditions of mild iodine deficiency. 2008;J Clin Endocrinol Metab 93:2616-2621.

[5] Stahl TJ. Radioimmunoassay and the hormones of thyroid function. 1975;Seminars in Nuclear Medicine, 5(3), 221-246.

[6] Taylor E and Heyland A. Evolution of thyroid hormone signaling in animals: Non-genomic and genomic modes of action. 2017;Molecular and Cellular Endocrinology, 459, 14-20.

[7] Venturi S and Venturi M. Evolution of dietary antioxidant defenses. 2007;European EpiMarker 11 (3): 1-12.

[8] Norris DO and Carr JA. The Hypothalamus-Pituitary-Thyroid Axis (HPT) of Non-Mammlian Vertebrates. Chapter 5. In: Vertebrate Endocrinology, fifth edition. 2013; San Diego, Academic Press. Pp 151-204.

[9] Watanabe Y and Weiss RE. Thyroid hormone action. In Martini L, editor. Encyclopedia of Endocrine Diseases. 2018;Elsevier pp. 452-462.

[10] Holzer G, Roux N, and Laudet V. Evolution of ligands, receptors and metabolizing enzymes of thyroid signaling. 2017;Molecular and Cellular Endocrinology. 459, 5-13.

[11] Heyland A, Price A, Bodnarova-Buganova M and Moroz LL. Thyroid hormone metabolism and peroxidase function in two non-chordate animals. 2006;J. Exp. Zool., 306B: 551-566.

[12] Wang S, Zhang S, Zhao B, and Lun L. Up-regulation of C/EBP by thyroid hormones: A case demonstrating the vertebrate-like thyroid hormone signaling pathway in amphioxus. 2009; Molecular and Cellular Endocrinology, 313(1-2): 57-63.

[13] Satoh N. The New Organizers Hypothesis for Chordate Origins. Chapter 7. In Chordate Origins and Evolution 2016;Academic Press. 97-120.

[14] Kluge B, Renault N, Rohr KB. Anatomical and molecular reinvestigation of lamprey endostyle development provides new insight into thyroid gland evolution. 2005;Dev Genes Evol 215:32-40.

[15] Gorbman, A. Hagfish Development. 1997;Zoological Science, 14(3): 375-390.

[16] Gerhart J. The deuterostome ancestor. 2006;Journal of Cellular Physiology, 209(3), 677-685.

[17] Simakov O, Kawashima T, Marlétaz F. *et al.* Hemichordate genomes and deuterostome origins. 2015;Nature 527, 459-465.

[18] Eales JG. Iodine metabolism and thyroid-related functions in organisms

lacking thyroid follicles: are thyroid hormones also vitamins? 1997;Proc. Soc. Exp. Bio. Med. 214:302-317.

[19] Heyland A and Moroz LL. Cross-kingdom hormonal signaling: an insight from thyroid hormone functions in marine larvae. 2005;The Journal of Experimental Biology 208, 4355-4361.

[20] Heyland A, Reitzel AM, and Hodin J. Thyroid hormones determine developmental mode in sand dollars (Echinodermata: Echinoidea). 2005;Evolution & Development 6:6, 382-392.

[21] Taylor E and Heyland A. Thyroid hormones accelerate initiation of skeletogenesis via MAPK (ERK1/2) in larval sea urchins (*S. purpuratus*). 2018;Frontiers in Endocrinology, 9, 439.

[22] Specker JL. Preadaptive role of thyroid hormones in larval and juvenile salmon: growth, the gut and evolutionary considerations. 1988;American Zoologist, 28 (2): 337-349.

[23] Brown CL, Urbinati E, Zhang W, Brown SB and McComb-Kobza M. Maternal thyroid and glucocorticoid hormone interactions in larval fish development, and their applications in aquaculture. 2014;Reviews in Fisheries Science and Aquaculture 22(3): 207-220.

[24] Heyland A, Hodin J, and Reitzel AM. Hormone signaling in evolution and development: a non-model system approach. 2005; BioEssays 27:64-75.

[25] Heyland A, Reitzel AM, Price DA, and Moroz LL. Endogenous thyroid hormone synthesis in facultative planktotrophic larvae of the sand dollar *C. rosaceus*: implications for the evolutionary loss of larval feeding. 2006;Evol Dev. 8(6): 568-579.

[26] Gonzalez P, Jiang JZ, and Lowe CJ. The development and metamorphosis of the indirect developing acorn worm *Schizocardium californicum* (Enteropneusta: Spengelidae). 2018;Frontiers in Zoology, 15(1).

[27] Blair JE, Hedges SB. Molecular phylogeny and divergence times of deuterostome animals, 2005;Molecular Biology and Evolution, 22 (11): 2275-2284.

[28] Barrington EJW, and Thorpe A. Comparative observations on lodine binding by *S. horsti* brambell and goodhart, and by the tunic of *Ciona intestinalis* (L). 1963;General and Comparative Endocrinology, 3(2), 166-175.

[29] Higa T, Fujiyama T, Scheuer PJ. Halogenated phenol and indole constituents of acorn worms. 1980;Comparative Biochemistry and Physiology Part B. 65 (3): 525-530,

[30] Fan T–P, Ting H-C, Yu J-K, and Su Y-H. Reiterative use of FGF signaling in mesoderm development during embryogenesis and metamorphosis in the hemichordate *Ptychodera flava*. 2018; BMC Evolutionary Biology, 18(1): 120.

[31] Koop D and Holland LZ The basal chordate amphioxus as a simple model for elucidating developmental mechanisms in vertebrates. 2008;Birth Defects Research Part C: Embryo Today: Reviews, 84: 175-187.

[32] Prowse TA, Byrne M. Evolution of yolk protein genes in the Echinodermata. 2012; Evol DevMar-Apr;14(2):139-51.

[33] Paris M, Brunet F, Markov GV, et al. The amphioxus genome enlightens the evolution of the thyroid hormone signaling pathway. Dev Genes Evol. 2008;**218**:667-680

[34] Röttinger E and Lowe CJ. Evolutionary crossroads in

developmental biology: hemichordates. 2012;*Development*; 139 (14): 2463-2475.

[35] Denver, R.J. 2008. Chordate metamorphosis: ancient control by iodothyronines. Current Biology, 18(13), R567-9. DOI: 10.1016/j.cub.2008.05.024.

[36] Holland LZ, Onai T. Early development of cephalochordates (Amphioxus). 2011;WIREs. Dev Biol. 2012;**1**:167-183

[37] Tagawa M and Brown CL. Entry of thyroid hormones into tilapia oocytes. 2001;Comparative Biochemistry and Physiology, B, 129, 605-611.

[38] Melianawati R, Pratiwi R, Puniawati N, and Astuti P. Effect of different kinds of live feed on thyroid structure of marine fish larvae coral trout *Plectropomus leopardus* (Lacepede, 1802). 2016;AIP Conference Proceedings 1755, 14005.

[39] Toledo JD, Golez MS, Doi M, and Ohno A. Use of copepod nauplii during early feeding stage of grouper *Epinephelus coioides*. 1999;Fisheries Science 65(3); 390-397.

[40] Burgess AI, Callan CK, Touse R, and Santos MD. Increasing survival and growth inlarval leopard coral grouper (*Plecotropomus leopardus*) using intensively cultured *Parvocalanus crassiostris* nauplii. 2019;Journal of the World Aquaculture Society 52:1 171-182.

[41] Brown, CL, Power DM, and Núñez JM. Disorders of Development in Fish. 2010;Pages 166-182. In: Leatherland, JK and Woo, PTK (Eds.), Fish Disease and Disorders, volume 2. Non-infectious disorders, second edition. CAB International Press, Wallingford, UK 400 Pp.

[42] Brown CL, Cochran M, Doroshov S, and Bern HA. Enhanced survival in striped bass fingerlings after maternal triiodothyronine treatment. 1988;Fish Physiol. Biochem., 7(1-6): 295-299.

[43] Brown CL, Doroshov S, Nunez J, Hadley C, Nishioka RS, and Bern HA. Maternal triiodothyronine injections cause increases in swimbladder inflation and survival rates in larval striped bass, *M. saxatilis*. 1988;J. Exp. Zool., 248: 168-176.

[44] Lam TJ. Hormones and egg / larval quality in fish. 1994;Journal of the World Aquaculture Society 25(1): 2-12.

[45] Molla MHR, M. T. Hasan MT, Jang WJ, Diaz CDS, Appenteng P, Marufchoni H, Jahan B, and Brown CL. Thyroid hormone-induced swim bladder and eye maturation are transduced by IGF-1 in zebrafish embryos. 2019;Aquaculture Research 00:1-9.

[46] Hu Y, Mauri A, Donahue J, Singh R, Acosta B, and McMenamin S. Thyroid hormone coordinates developmental trajectories but does not underlie developmental truncation in danionins. 2019;Dev Dyn 248(11):1144-1154.

[47] Deal CK and Volkoff H. The role of the thyroid axis in fish. 2020;Front. Endocrinol 06; https://doi.org/10.3389/fendo.2020.596585

[48] Afarinesh MR, Shafiei F, Sabzalizadeh M, Haghpanah T, Taheri M, Parsania S, Golshan F, and Sheibani V. Effect of mild and chronic neonatal hypothyroidism on sensory information processing in a rodent model: A behavioral and electrophysiological study. 2020;Brain Res Bull. 155:29-36. doi: 10.1016/j.brainresbull.2019.11.015. Epub 2019 Nov 28. PMID: 31786270.

[49] Singleman C and Holtzman G. Growth and maturation in the Zebrafish, *Danio rerio*: A staging tool for teaching and research. 2014;Zebrafish. 11(4): 396-406. doi: 10.1089/zeb.2014.0976.

[50] Reddy PK and Lam TJ. Effect of thyroid hormones on the morphogenesis and growth of larvae and fry of telescopic-eye black goldfish, *Carassius auratus*. 1992;Aquaculture, 107: 383-394.

[51] Reddy PK, and Lam TJ. Role of thyroid hormones in tilapia larva (*Oreochromis mossambicus*): I. Effects of the hormones and an antithyroid drug on yolk absorption, growth and development. 1992;Fish Physiol. Biochem., 9(5-6): 473-485.

[52] Shubin N. Some Assembly Required. Decoding Four Billion Years of Life, From Ancient Fossils to DNA. 2020;Pantheon Books, NY. 267 Pp.

[53] Wilcoxon JS, Nadolski GJ, Samarut J, Chassande O, and Redei EE. Behavioral inhibition and impaired spatial learning and memory in hypothyroid mice lacking thyroid hormone receptor alpha. 2007;Behav Brain Res. 177(1):109-116. doi:10.1016/j.bbr.2006.10.030

[54] American Thyroid Association. Hypothyroidism: A Booklet for Patients and Their Families. 2019;https://www.thyroid.org/wp-content/uploads/patients/brochures/Hypothyroidism_web_booklet.pdf. Accessed August 20, 2021.

[55] Kurokawa T, Kagawa H, Ohta H, Tanaka H, Okuzawa K, and Hirose K. Development of digestive organs and feeding ability in larvae of Japanese eel (*A. japonica*). 1995;Can. J. Fish. Aquat. Sci. 52: 1030-1036.

[56] Adachi S, Ijiri S, Kazeto Y, Yamauchi K. Oogenesis in the Japanese Eel, *A. japonica*. In: Aida K., Tsukamoto K., Yamauchi K. (editors) Eel Biology. 2003;Springer. Tokyo.

[57] Brown CL and Kim BG Combined application of cortisol and triiodothyronine in the culture of larval marine finfish. 1995;Aquaculture 135(1-3): 79-86.

[58] Kim BG and Brown CL. Interaction of cortisol and thyroid hormone in the larval development of Pacific threadfin. 1997;American Zoologist 37: 470-481.

[59] Kim BG, Divakaran S, Brown CL, and Ostrowski AC. Comparative digestive enzyme ontogeny in two marine larval fishes: Pacific threadfin (*Polydactylus sexfilis*) and bluefin trevally (*Caranx melampygus*). 2001;Fish Physiology and Biochemistry 24: 225-241.

[60] Daher R, Yazbeck T, Jaoude JB, and Abboud B. Consequences of dysthyroidism on the digestive tract and viscera. 2009;World J Gastroenterol 15(23): 2834-2838.

[61] Kjorsvic E, Mangor-Jensen A, and Holmefjord J. Egg quality in fishes. 1990;Advances in Marine Biology 26:71-113.

[62] O'Sullivan RJ, Aykanat T, Johnston SE, Rogan G, Poole R, Prodohl PA, de Eyto E, Primmer CR, McGinnity P, and Reed TE. Captive-bred Atlantic salmon relesed into the wild have fewer offspring than wild-bred fish and decrease population productivity. 2020;Proceedings of the Royal Society B: 287 1937.

[63] Fontaine R, Affaticiati P, Yamamoto K, Jolly C, Bureau C, Baloche S, Gonnet F, Vernier P, Dufour S, and Pasqualini C. Dopamine inhibits reproduction in female zebrafish (*D. rerio*) via three pituitary D2 receptor subtypes. 2013;Neuroendocrinology 154(2): 807-818.

[64] Singh K, Dutt S, Ali M, and Biswas RK. Use of dopamine antagonists on induced spawning of Indian major carps. 1996;Journal of the Indian Fisheries Association Proc. Nat. Symp. Aquacrops 75-84.

[65] Solbakken JS, Berntessen MHG, Norberg B, and Hamre K. Different iodine and thyroid hormone levels

between Atlantic halibut larvae fed wild zooplankton or *Artemia* from first exogenous feeding until post metamorphosis. 2005;Journal of Fish Biology 61:1341-1362.

[66] Garrido S, Ben-Hamadou R, Santos AMP, Ferreira S, Teodósio MA, Cotano U, Irigoien X, Peck MA, Saiz E, and Ré P. Born small, die young: Intrinsic, size-selective mortality in marine larval fish. 2105;Sci Rep 5, 17065. https://doi.org/10.1038/srep17065

[67] McComb DM, Gelsleichter J, Manire CA, and Brown C.L. Comparative thyroid hormone concentration in maternal serum and yolk of the bonnethead shark (*Sphyrna tiburo*) from two sites along the coast of Florida. 2005;General and Comparative Endocrinology 144(2): 167-173.

[68] Plohman JC, Dick TA, and Eales JG. Thyroid of lake sturgeon, *Acipenser fulvescens*. I. Hormone levels in blood and tissues. 2002;Gen Comp Endocrinol 125(1):47-55. doi: 10.1006/gcen.2001.7733.

[69] Kuhn ER, Mol K, and Darras VM. Peripheral deiodination of thyroid hormones: Biological significance. 1994;Neth. J. Zool., 45(1-2):135-139.

[70] Denver RJ. Stress hormones mediate developmental plasticity in vertebrates with complex life cycles. 2021;Neurobiology of Stress 14: 100301.

[71] De Jesus EG, Inui Y, and Hirano T. Cortisol enhances the stimulating action of thyroid hormones on dorsal fin-ray resorption of flounder larvae in vitro. 1990;Gen. Comp. Endocrinol., 79: 167-173.

[72] Pataueg AJ. A Theoretical basis for the integration of developmental and thermoregulatory roles of thyroid hormones in vertebrata. 2021;Master of Science in Fisheries Thesis, World Fisheries University, Pukyong National University, Busan. S. Korea.

Chapter 9

Molecular Mechanisms of Glucose Uptake Regulation in Thyroid Cancer

Shabnam Heydarzadeh, Ali Asghar Moshtaghie, Maryam Daneshpour and Mehdi Hedayati

Abstract

Common capabilities of thyroid malignant cells are accelerating metabolism and increasing glucose uptake to optimize energy supply for growth. In tumor cells, keeping the power load required for cell survival is essential and glucose transporters are capable of promoting this task. GLUT-1 and GLUT3 are promising goals for the development of anti-cancer strategies. The lack of oncosuppressors has dominant effect on the membrane expression of GLUT1 and glucose uptake. Overexpression of hypoxia-inducing factors, in thyroid cancer, modulates the expression of some glucose transporter genes. Although the physiology of the thyroid gland has been excellently explained, metabolic regulation in thyroid cancer is inevitable. In this section, we investigated the proliferation pathways of pivotal regulators and signal molecules around GLUT regulation in thyroid cancer, including PTEN, p53, MicroRNA, iodide, BRAF, HIF-1, PI3K-Akt, TSH, c-Myc, and AMPK. Impaired energy regulation and cell metabolism are the most critical symptoms of most cancers. As a result, understanding the mechanisms of glucose transport in the normal and pathological tissues of the thyroid may be very crucial and offer tremendous insights into the science of analysis and remedy of thyroid disease.

Keywords: thyroid cancer, glucose uptake, regulator, glucose transporter

1. Introduction

In glucose metabolism, glucose transport in the plasma membrane, known as the rate-limiting step, is mediated by carriers belonging to the facilitative glucose transporter (GLUT) and the sodium-coupled glucose co-transporter (SGLT) proteins families. While SGLTs require energy to perform the task of glucose transport, GLUT allows glucose to be transported below its concentration gradient without energy dependence [1]. GLUT1 is one of the fourteen GLUT isoforms that have a strong affinity for glucose and express unusual expression of plasma membranes [2, 3]. High expression of GLUT1 is positively correlated with proliferation index and is equivalent to malignant characteristic. In this case, there are poor foresight in different types of cancer, including prostate [4], thyroid [5, 6], colon [7, 8], melanoma [9], liver [10], breast [11, 12], and ovary [13, 14].

Almost many cancer cells change cellular metabolism due to high proliferation rates, which can lead to a stressful metabolic phenotype. Tumor cells are able to alter metabolism from oxidative to glycolytic phenotype. This effect is called Warburg, which is a specific metabolic feature of the tumor and a major metabolic feature. Research on tumor metabolism suggests that rapid cell proliferation, tumor progression, and resistance to cell death should be maintained by altering cellular metabolism in which glycolysis and glutaminolysis are regulated [15]. Glucose transfer occurs in neoplastic cells across the plasma membrane, the first step in limiting the rate of glucose metabolism. There is evidence that a decrease in GLUT1 can suppress cell proliferation, so regulating glucose transporter expression and activity has a significant effect on glucose supply in cancer cells [16]. Several studies have shown the immunohistochemistry of GLUT 1 in cancer cell research [17–19]. High expression of GLUT1 on plasma membranes is related to exactly the same degree of differentiation. Also, the biological invasion of thyroid cancer (TC) is commonly occurred in ATC compared to other different types. GLUT1 is located on the plasma membrane and their expression can be assessed by using PET [20].

One hallmark of cancer cells; especially TC cells are showing high glucose uptake than the normal thyroid samples. Tumor cells regenerate their metabolism by increasing the transportation of glucose to promote cell survival. Malignant cells increase the transportation of glucose through the cell membrane by inducing a family of facilitative glucose-transporting proteins (GLUTs) that are highly classifiable in terms of tissue-specific distribution and different tendencies to glucose and different transport capacities. In most cases, thyroid cancer cells often show overexpression of the GLUT1 and GLUT3 proteins that respond to hypoxia. Malignant cells are typically less able to utilize oxidative metabolism, but aerobic glycolysis is rapidly increased and oxidative phosphorylation remains constant. Increased glycolysis is the main source of energy in cancer cells, but due to the lower energy function in the glycolytic pathway, malignant cells increase the rate of glucose transport in the plasma membrane to compensate for the energy obtained [21–25].

Recently, the relationship between tumor differentiation and glucose metabolism in thyroid cancer has been investigated. The metabolic profile of glucose is differently related to differentiation in well-differentiated and poorly differentiated thyroid cancer. During Suh H. Y. et al. studies based on genetic mutation, the metabolic profile of TC cells was not simply linked with differentiation. The expression of GLUT had an opposite relationship with differentiation in TC. Glycolysis enhancing had a positive relationship with the well-differentiated TC, and on the other hand, showed a negative relationship with poorly differentiated TC. In the papillary type of TC, glycolysis signature showed a positive correlation with differentiation rate, while GLUT signature had a negative correlation with differentiation rate. On the other hand, in the poorly differentiated type of TC, both GLUT and glycolysis showed a negative relationship with the differentiation rate. Their results were in agreement with previous investigations because poorly differentiated type with overexpression of GLUT requires more glucose uptake. In general, it is considered that the relationship between the differentiation and glycolysis may follow a U-shape pattern. The results of different rates for GLUT and glycolysis in PTC were the BRAFV600E mutation status. The PTC cells containing BRAFV600E mutation had high GLUT signature and low glycolysis signature than PTC cells that did not contain BRAFV600E mutation [26].

It is reported that GLUT1, GLUT3, GLUT4, and GLUT10 are expressed in all thyroid parenchymal cells, without attention to their histological status. GLUT1 is more expressed in thyroid cancer tissues than in normal and benign samples obtained from the same patient. Other GLUTs have not been reported to be altered in comparison to GLUT1 in the same patient's pathological tissues. These results indicated that GLUT1 is theoretically responsible for the observed increase in glucose uptake during carcinogenesis [27, 28]. Overexpression of hexokinase I and increased intracellular glucose phosphorylation in thyroid tumors have been shown to be a signal of tumor invasion. The degree of tumor differentiation in thyroid cancer is consistent with the expression of GLUTs. While poorly differentiated types (anaplastic) have a high expression of GLUT (mainly GLUT1), in contrast, well-differentiated tumors (follicular and papillary) often have a weak expression of GLUT1. GLUT-3 has been reported to be predominant in papillary thyroid cancer [20, 29]. Based on the results of the research, there was a significant expression of GLUT1, GLUT3, and GLUT4 in the cytoplasm and/or membrane of PTC. In PTC cells, GLUT3 and GLUT4 expression pattern were higher than GLUT1 one [30].

The expression of GLUT1 and GLUT3 induced by hypoxia is not similar in benign and malignant thyroid tissues as well as non-neoplastic samples. The dissimilarity in expression levels of GLUT1 and GLUT3 are related to the sample histology. The hypoxia-induced GLUT1 and 3 have a role in the progress of PTC and may be contributed to the panel of significant markers of thyroid cancer. High expressions of GLUT1 and GLUT3 proteins showed a direct relationship with high levels of GLUT1 and GLUT3 mRNA in similar samples of TC. In spite of that, in some of the neoplasm samples, the GLUT1 or GLUT3 band and also mRNA levels were very low. The best interpretation for these detections is the influence of the hypoxia-induced GLUTs by the cancer cell microenvironment and oxygen-related transcription factors [31].

Unusual expression of GLUT proteins is controlled by multiple signal transduction pathways, including the phosphoinositide 3-kinase (PI3K) / AKT pathway [32]. In the thyroid glands, AMPK plays an important physiological role in the uptake of thyroid iodide and can play a role in carcinogenesis. It is recently found that in TC cells, AMPK can increase glucose uptake through the inducing of GLUT 1 and hexokinase (HK) activity [33, 34]. Lack of PTEN expression can lead to the AKT pathway inhibition that was linked with superficial expression of GLUT1 and the possibility of TC diagnosis by FDG-PET [35].

Thyroidectomy and radioactive iodine therapy are common treatments for patients with thyroid cancer but often are not more effective. Recent advances in molecular therapies aimed to understand the molecular pathogenesis of thyroid cancer were promising in the development of early detection and appropriate treatment strategies for thyroid cancer. This is mainly due to the detection of molecular alterations [36]. Although the physiological function of the thyroid gland is well established, its metabolic compatibility is unclear, especially in thyroid cancer. This review argues for recent significant advances and key factors, including inhibiting or stimulating glucose uptake in thyroid cancer that may be useful for future therapeutic purposes in this disease.

2. Targeting glucose transportation in cancer cells

It has been well known from the time of Warburg's hypothesis that cancer cells were found to show the high need for energy and metabolism. It has been reported that almost 90% of cancers showed high glucose metabolism. In addition, these cells, despite having oxygen, can reduce the oxidative phosphorylation pathway and are in favor of the pyruvate conversion to lactate. ATP synthesis is not the top priority of the upregulation of glucose transport. Glycolysis is approximately 18 times more efficient than the oxidative phosphorylation process, so cancer cells need more glucose uptake into cells to compensate for low ATP production [37–39]. Although the Warburg effect was observed more than 80 years ago, its

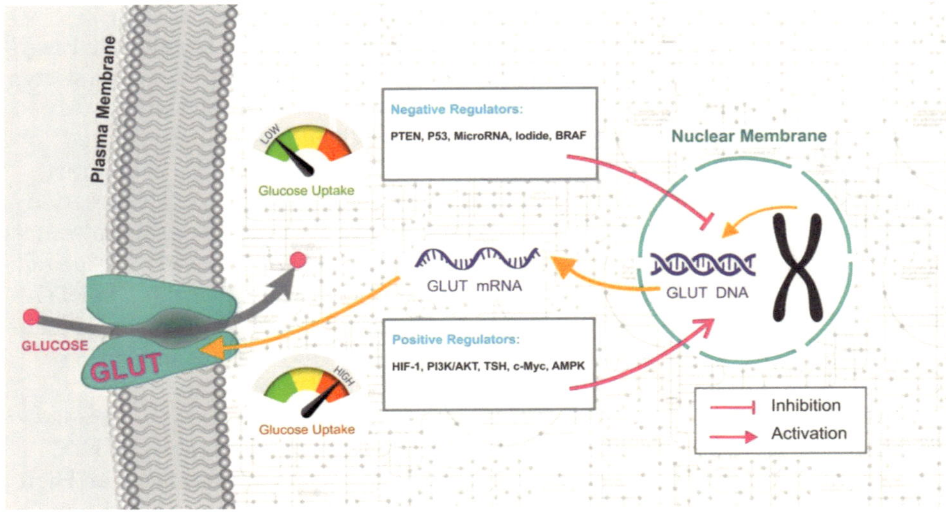

Figure 1.
Positive and negative regulators of glucose uptake.

interpretation is still argumentative and evolving. Cancer cells do not tend to convert all of the glucose from regulated transport into pyruvate, but rather turn some of the metabolic mediators of glucose into the pentose phosphate pathway (PPP), which is a metabolic pathway, branched off from glycolysis that provides metabolic intermediates for the synthesis of biomass [40–42]. At present, clinical and basic science studies have shown that the Warburg effect is a potential and intelligent cancer research area [43]. Targeting glucose metabolism and transport has been suggested as a useful target for cancer therapeutic intervention [39, 44, 45]. Glycolytic switching in cancer, in addition to greater potential for invasion and metastasis [46], increases the susceptibility of cancer to external interference due to their greater dependence on aerobic glycolysis [47–49]. The discovery of GLUT inhibitors may indicate the development of drugs that can be used as anticancer agents, possibly in addition to conventional chemotherapy or new immunotherapies for further study [50]. There is strong evidence that the expression, activity, and intracellular movement of GLUTs as malignant biomarkers are regulated by different signaling molecules and pathways. In this study, we investigated the proliferation pathways of key positive and negative regulators and signal molecules including PI3K-Akt, HIF-1, MicroRNA, PTEN, AMPK, BRAF, c-Myc, TSH, iodide, and p53, which consist of GLUT regulation in thyroid cancer cells (**Figure 1**).

3. Negative regulation of glucose uptake

3.1 PTEN

PTEN (phosphatase and tensin homolog deleted on chromosome 10) is known as a protein and lipid phosphatase that suppresses tumors and negatively regulates cell growth and metabolism. This gene is often mutated in many advanced human cancers [51]. PTEN expression and activity may be affected by intragenic mutations or epigenetic silencing and post-translational changes. Histone de-acetylation is one of the factors that shut down the genetic process that affects PTEN expression. Researches have shown that inhibition of histone deacetylase can save PTEN expression and reduce the AKT pathway as well as glucose transport [52]. Loss of PTEN as tumor suppressor gene, possessing an inhibitory role on PI3K / AKT signaling pathway, has also been involved in FTC progression.

Scientific researchers have identified the relationship between plasma PTEN levels and sporadic PTC and their involvement as biomarkers. The observation of PTEN promoter hypermethylation in approximately 50% of PTCs and 100% of FTCs proposes that it may have a contribution to thyroid carcinogenesis [53, 54]. Glucose uptake signaling pathways that occurred during thyroid cancer is poorly recognized since now. Genetic manipulations showed that PTEN as an oncosuppressor agent have participation in GLUT1 expression and glucose uptake in TC cells. Lack of PTEN expression can block the AKT pathway and is associated with the possibility of rapid detection of thyroid cancer by FDG-PET. PTEN binds to SNX27 and prevents it from accessing the VPS26 retromer complex, thus blocking GLUT1 glucose transporter recycling to the plasma membrane, leading to impaired cellular glucose uptake [55, 56]. PTEN can also affect glucose metabolism by dephosphorylating the insulin-1 receptor substrate, thus inhibiting insulin signals and insulin growth factors that are also associated with glucose metabolism [52].

The PI3k class I (PI3KC1) -AKT pathway and AKT downstream effector AS160 (GTPase rab activator) are involved in GLUT1 cell surface exposure in thyroid cancer cells [57, 58]. PTEN lipid phosphatase activity is a determinant of PTEN inhibitory action on the AKT pathway which antagonizes the activation of the AKT pathway. This can reduce the availability of phosphatidylinositol [3–5] -tris phosphate (PIP3), which is a phosphate donor for AKT phosphorylation. This prevents the expression of GLUT1 in the plasma membrane and ultimately the anti-cancer function. It has not been revealed whether PTEN protein phosphatase activity also affects PI3K activity and GLUT1 regulation on plasma membranes. It has been reported that even the AKT pathway can be regulated by PTEN through protein phosphatase activity [52].

3.2 P53

Environmental, genetic, and hormonal factors are the main roots of human malignancy incidence [59], among which genetic factors indicate an extraordinary role in carcinogenesis. Different types of incidence and progression of thyroid cancer are characterized by the gradual accumulation of somatic mutations and/or gene rearrangement with different frequencies and properties [60, 61]. Today, the absence of p53 family members indicates the pathogenesis of poorly differentiated thyroid tumors. Inactive P53 is a genetic variant that distinguishes anaplastic thyroid cancer from well-differentiated thyroid cancer. The p53 mutation usually occurs in undifferentiated thyroid tumors (50–80% in ATCs) [60, 62]. In addition, recent studies have shown that genetic variation of p53 is distinguished in 40% of papillary thyroid cancer and 22% of follicular thyroid cancer [63, 64].

PTEN and P53 play a key role in driving GLUT1 in the plasma membrane. They are key regulators of glucose metabolism and autophagy, which are the most common deleted or mutated suppressors in human cancer [65–67]. Expression of PTEN and P53 can be the cause of glucose uptake and glycolytic enzymes inhibition, stimulation of apoptotic cell death, and mitochondrial oxidation induction, accordingly counteracting with the Warburg effect. They block the PI3k-AKT–mTOR signaling, so it can regulate cell growth. TC cells with an unusual expression of PTEN or p53 are more likely to consume glucose. These two regulators have been shown to stimulate tumor cells to overcome hypoxia-induced metabolic stress and glucose depletion. It also inhibits caspase-dependent apoptosis, autophagy, promotes cell migration, and invasion [68–70].

Point mutations in p53, which occurred in the domain of its binding to DNA, have been associated with malignancy and have abolished its inhibitory activity on the transcriptional activity of GLUTs. Among the GLUTs, GLUT1 and GLUT4 gene promoters are the dominant types that are affected by the P53 mutation in a dose-dependent manner. This results in an increase in glycometabolism and cellular energy, which is known to facilitate tumor cell growth. P53 has shown a significant inhibitory effect on GLUT4 compared to GLUT1. This may be due to the fact that GLUT1 is a general "housekeeping" transporter of glucose, whereas GLUT4 is a tissue-specific and insulin-sensitive glucose carrier [71, 72].

3.3 MicroRNA

MicroRNAs (miRNAs) are classified into oncogenic and tumor suppressor miRNAs. Onco-miRNAs are elevated in human cancers that inhibit cell growth and apoptosis, whereas tumor-suppressive miRNAs are downregulated in human cancers and can prevent cancer progression [73–75]. MiRNAs are non-coding, evolutionarily conserved RNAs that bind to the 3'-UTRs of messenger RNAs and are referred to as negative regulators following transcription [76]. Recent research suggests that a TC invasion is frequently characterized by a lack of miRNA regulation. MiR-146b, MiR-221, and MiR-222 are invasive PTC predictors [77–79].

MiR-718, which is a known negative regulator of proliferation, metastasis, and glucose metabolism, exhibits anti-cancer activity in PTC. MiR-718 can diminish the intensity of PTC cells by inhibiting the Akt–mTOR messaging pathway. MiR-718 expression was significantly decreased in malignant samples compared to normal papillary thyroid tissue. Due to the study of miR-718's influence on PDPK1, p-Akt, Akt, and p-mTOR, it was determined that p-Akt and p-mTOR were reduced following PTC treatment with MiR-718. MicroRNA was found to have a detrimental influence on the primary stages of the Akt–mTOR signaling pathway. It follows the regulation of the proliferation, migration, and invasion of PTC cells. The Akt–mTOR signaling pathway has been shown to play an important role in tumor cell glucose metabolism and phenotypic severity. Overexpression of MiR-718 has a significant effect on reducing energy production in PTC cells. Taken together, these results suggest that microRNAs such as miR-718 negatively regulate metabolic activity in thyroid cancer cells [80, 81].

MiR-125a-5p has been demonstrated to act as a tumor suppressor and glucose metabolism regulator in a range of malignancies, most notably TC [82]. Due to the fact that lactate is the end product of glycolysis in tumor cells and can be easily measured, its detection shows the rate of glucose metabolism. MiR-125a-5p reduces lactate synthesis, ATP production, and glucose uptake in TC cells, resulting in a blockage of glycolysis, decreased migration, and cell invasion. The MiR-125a-5p/CD147 axis has been suggested to possibly play an important role in the aerobic glycolysis of thyroid cancer cells. Because GLUT1, HK2, MCT1, and MCT4 are important glycolysis-related proteins, their expression levels are significantly regulated by the miR-125a-5p/CD147 axis (**Figure 2**) [83, 84].

3.4 Iodide

Iodide is responsible for regulating the activity of thyroid cells. The number of glucose carriers in the plasma membrane can be reduced by the iodine auto-regulation function of iodine. In fact, it not only affects glucose metabolism through the oxidation pathway but also through an inhibitory effect on the glucose-facilitating transport system. Iodide is able to inhibit TSH-induced stimulation of glucose transport. The role

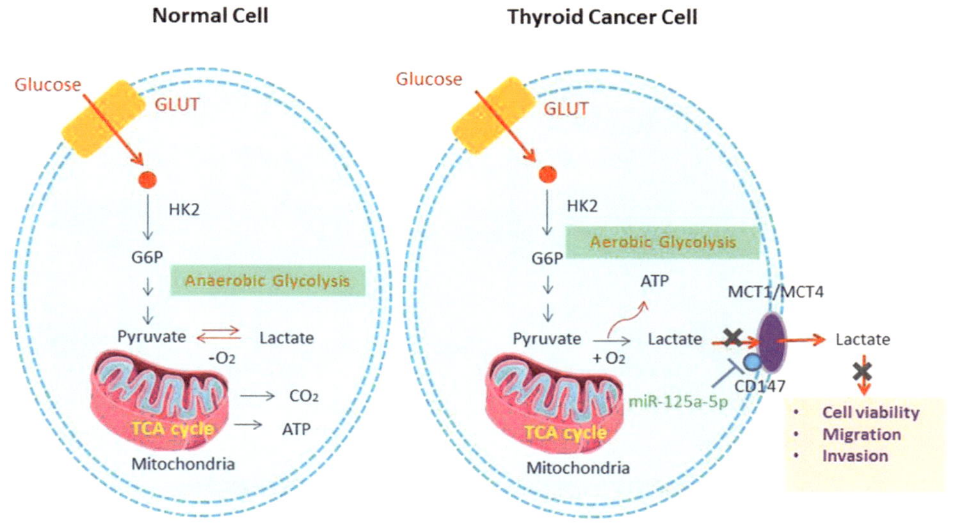

Figure 2.
Metabolic diversity between the Normal and cancer cells of the thyroid. Normal cells primarily consume glucose through the oxidation of pyruvate to CO_2 by the TCA cycle. TC cells convert most glucose to lactate, regardless of the availability of O_2, through the overexpression of some special glucose metabolism-related proteins. MiR-125a-5p blocks the effect of CD147 on lactate transporters such as MCT1/MCT4 that is resulted in low viability, migration, and invasion of TC cells.

of thyroid hormone in the automatic regulation of iodine has also been recognized, but T3 and T4 do not block glucose transportation. Iodide can block the Vmax of glucose transport without any interference on Km. Therefore; iodine has not any function through the affinity to glucose, but can result in a low number of available transporter sites. As a consequence, the inhibitory role of iodine on glucose uptake in thyroid tissues may be crucial in both physiological and pathological status, as well as metabolism and nucleic acid mediators [85]. Poor differentiation is associated with upregulation of GLUT1 in TC cells that led to severe malignant biological phenotypes. The dedifferentiation process of FTC cells is associated with iodine loss. In addition, it was reported that thyroid malignancies become more eager for glucose during the dedifferentiation. This inverse communication between iodine and glucose (measured by ^{18}FFDG PET/CT) was determined as the flip-flop phenomenon (**Figure 3**). This pattern is distinguished in different patients as well as in different locations of the tumor in one patient [20, 86].

3.5 BRAF

BRAF is a cytoplasmic serine–threonine protein kinase that shows a crucial role in thyroid carcinogenesis. Finding of BRAF mutation as a common change in TC is important knowledge. The BRAF mutation may initiate the transition of PTC to ATC [87]. The differentiated thyroid cancers with mutant-type BRAF show more levels of GLUT-1 than those with wild-type BRAF. These results suggest that tumor cells with BRAF genetic variants may have higher uptake of 18F-FDG.

It has been recognized that there is a link between mutant BRAF and downstream stimulation of MAPK. The c-Myc linkage targets HIF-1a that resulted to high glucose metabolism [88]. The incidence of BRAF V600E mutations may participate in glycolytic phenotypes associated with overexpression of GLUT1. In this case, GLUT1 is the target of the RAF / MEK / ERK activated pathway. This contribution leads to cancer cells growth [89, 90]. BRAF and MAP/ERK kinase inhibitors give the assurance in cancer therapy linked with BRAF mutations [91].

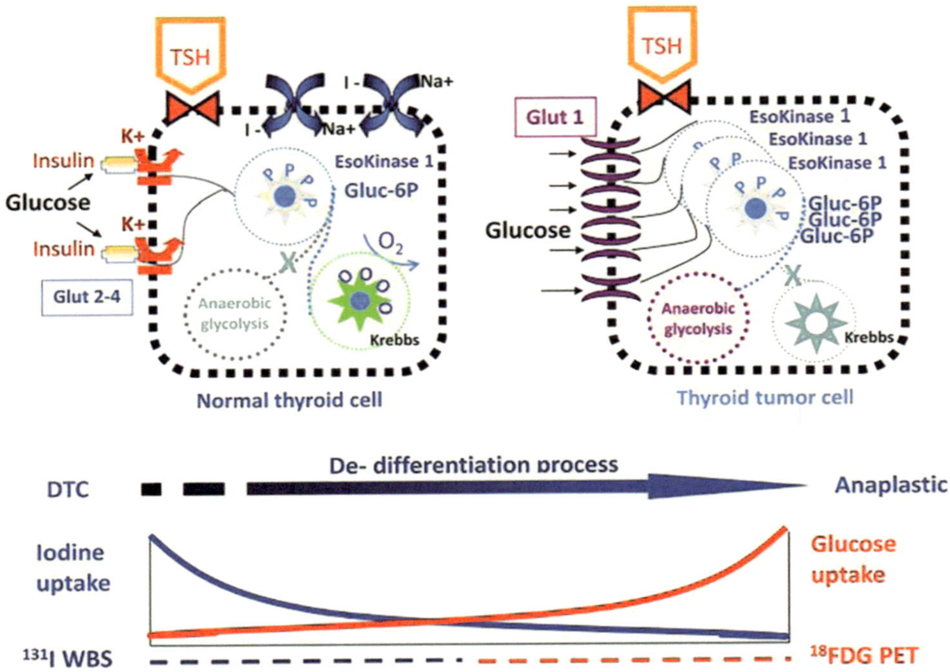

Figure 3.
Molecular basis of flipflop phenomenon.

4. Positive regulation of glucose uptake

4.1 HIF-1

Hypoxia is an important feature of invasive malignancies that causes malignant phenotypes and activates the physiological adaptation of cancer cells. This helps the tumor to survive and also to progress the diseases. Examples of this adaptation for cancer cells include the glucose transporter 1 gene (GLUT1), which increases glucose uptake for glycolysis [92]. Evidences suggest that the high rate of HIF-1a signaling observed in many tumors can lead to tumor metastasis, poor prognosis, or therapy. It is important to note that HIF-1a signaling is induced by low oxygen uptake as well as by oncogenic stimulation through abnormal growth mediators or lack of tumor suppressors [93]. The level of HIF-1a protein and the upregulation of reporter gene activity is equal to the increase in GLUT1 levels. HIF-1a expression is increased in FTC-133 cells with PTEN mutation. There is an important correlation between PI3K/AKT and HIF-1a that may be particularly associated with disease progression in thyroid cancer [86].

There is no sign of HIF-1α expression in normal thyroid tissue, but it is highly expressed in the most invasive differential thyroid cancers. In PTC, MTC, and FTC, overexpression of HIF-1 is associated with poor prognosis and distant metastasis [15, 93]. Thyroid hormones can activate the PI3K and MAPK signal cascades. In addition, thyroid hormones have the task of directly regulating HIF-1α expression by stimulating these signal transduction pathways. A TRβ mutation binds to the PI3K-regulatory subunit p85α following high signaling of PI3K and causes thyroid tumorigenesis, which may result in high HIF-1α expression [93].

HIF-1 contributes to the Warburg effect by increasing glycolysis. It is performed through the stimulation of all glycolytic enzymes, as well as increasing their substrates affinity [83]. HIF-1 also can increase the GLUTs level and decrease mitochondrial metabolism, which may be important in inhibiting ROS production and protecting cancer cells from death [94, 95]. HIF-1 has been suggested to help the Warburg effect by stimulating a number of glycolysis-mediated genes [96, 97], including GLUT1 and GLUT3, which contain hypoxia-reactive elements (HRE) in their promoters [98, 99].

In addition, HIF-1 can show a direct effect on the expression of all 12 enzymes required for glycolysis, or glucose and lactate transporters. These factors showed high expression in TC. In general, these results suggest that TC cells showed the Warburg effect by altering the energy supply by increasing the glycolysis pathway and decreasing mitochondrial function [100]. The close association of HIF-1α with metabolic pathways may be a welcome goal for better treatment of thyroid cancer [92].

4.2 PI3K/AKT

The phosphatidylinositol 3-kinase (PI3K)-Akt pathway is a family of growth factor-activated lipid and protein kinases that are involved in the regulation of growth and survival processes [101]. The PI3K/Akt pathway was initially associated with thyroid cancer due to the proclivity of patients with Cowden's syndrome to develop thyroid cancer. Due to the fact that Akt phosphorylates a vast number of downstream cytoplasmic and nuclear mediators, it is involved in the regulation of a variety of activities, including glucose metabolism. Increased PI3K/Akt expression appears to be connected with a poor prognosis in a variety of malignancies. Although the PI3K/Akt pathway plays a crucial role in endocrine malignancies, it has received less attention than other types of tumors [102].

The PI3K/Akt pathway mediates increased glucose uptake and overexpression of GLUT in cancers and is also involved in stimulating glucose transport in normal insulin-responsive tissues to increase glucose uptake [103]. PTEN functions as a tumor suppressor by blocking the PI3K/AKT pathway. The absence of this inhibitor can result in enhanced PI3K signaling, which can result in carcinogenesis. In malignancies, overactivation of Akt in the absence of a suppressor may result in enhanced glucose absorption. The serine/threonine kinase Akt, which is downstream of PI3K, is implicated in mediating the Warburg effect and triggering the expression of GLUTs such as GLUT1, GLUT3, and GLUT5 [101, 103–105]. It also acts as a regulator of GLUT4 transport around the plasma membrane, which facilitates glucose transport [103].

The effect of oncogenes on the metabolic change of cells to maintain cell proliferation is a major aspect of thyroid tumors [106]. In many tumors, activation of the PI3K / AKT pathway may be associated with mutations in RAS [107] leading to increased glycolysis flux [108, 109]. The PI3K / AKT pathway in the transfer of the GLUT1 cytoplasm to the plasma membrane in thyroid cells is very significant [15, 32]. According to the list of somatic mutations in cancer, PI3K/Akt pathway mutations are more prevalent in follicular and anaplastic thyroid tumors but are less prevalent in papillary thyroid cancer.

PI3K/Akt signaling has been implicated in thyroid carcinogenesis in animal studies. Thyroid cancer incidence is dramatically reduced in patients with Akt deficiency. Additionally, there is considerable evidence that AKT activation occurs in human thyroid cancer [96, 110, 111]. Numerous medicines targeting the PI3K/Akt signaling pathways are now being explored in phase I to III clinical studies. Temsirolimus and everolimus have been discovered to be very effective in the treatment of thyroid cancer [112].

4.3 TSH

TSH is an abbreviation for Thyroid Stimulating Hormone, a hormone that plays a critical role in the regulation of the activity and metabolism of normal thyroid cells. Its stimulation increases glucose metabolism to enhance iodide transport and thyroid hormone synthesis (T3 and T4) [15]. Increased glucose uptake in tumor cells may reflect changes in gene expression or increased transmission to the cell surface. According to study, thyroid cells enhance their glucose absorption in response to thyroid-stimulating hormone activity. TSH, on the other hand, does not appear to have a substantial effect on GLUT gene expression, indicating that TSH alters glucose uptake through shifting/transferring GLUT rather than boosting GLUT gene expression [27]. TSH significantly increased the cellular absorption of 2-deoxy-D-glucose and the glucose transport tracer 3-O-methyl-D-glucose, both of which were labeled with carbon-14. Additionally, it has been demonstrated that enhanced glucose transfer may be a factor in increased GLUT1 transfer to the thyroid cell surface. These findings may help for explanation of the increased absorption of FDG with high TSH [113].

TSH can promote glucose absorption in normal thyroid tissue. TSH stimulation has an effect on adenylate cyclase, increasing the levels of cAMP. The results indicated an increase in glucose metabolism in a well-differentiated rat cell line FRTL-5. TSH-induced increase in 18F-FDG accumulation is dependent on phosphatidylinositol-3-kinase (PI3-kinase) in FRTL-5 cells. TSH or cAMP influence glucose absorption in thyroid cancer cells. This is depending on the activity of the PI3-kinase triggered by the mutant K-ras oncogene. TSH-induced glucose uptake was studied in ML-1 and FRTL-5 cell lines. This diversity is due to the clinical heterogeneity of various tumor morphologies and the degree of differentiation of tumor cells. Increased PI3-kinase activity, which may be induced by oncogenes such as mutant Ras, is responsible for glucose uptake in dedifferentiated thyroid cancer, indicating possible pathogenesis for thyroid malignancies (**Figure 4**) [107, 108, 114].

TSH affects FDG absorption in a time and concentration-dependent manner through TSH receptors. At high TSH levels, glucose absorption is enhanced in well-differentiated thyroid carcinomas, which are typically still sensitive to TSH. TSH receptor messenger RNA expression in thyroid malignancies has been linked to the degree of differentiation, and poorly differentiated thyroid carcinomas may lack TSH receptors [115, 116]. Thyroid malignancies have been shown to contain somatic mutations in the TSH receptor gene as well as other CAMP cascade alterations, thus even when the TSH receptor is expressed, malignant tissue may respond to TSH stimulation differently than normal tissue. As a result, not all thyroid tumors are likely to accumulate FDG in TSH stimulation to the same degree as normal thyroid tissue [113]. The link between FDG uptake and TSH levels is of therapeutic relevance and might lead to new treatments. The link between FDG uptake and TSH levels is clinically significant and may result in significant misinterpretations in therapeutic studies [114].

4.4 c-Myc

c-MYC, a proto-oncogene, is a known cause of cancer. Myc has been demonstrated to directly influence glucose metabolism genes. The glucose transporter GLUT1, hexokinase 2 (HK2), phosphofructokinase (PFKM), and enolase 1 are the most essential of these [117–119]. Recently, it was demonstrated that glucose metabolism inhibitors targeting MYC inhibited the expression of GLUT-1, LDH-A, and MCT1 in cancer cell lines, coupled with lower MYC activity, hence inhibiting cell proliferation and tumor formation. Is it [120]. Myc controls the expression of genes involved in the

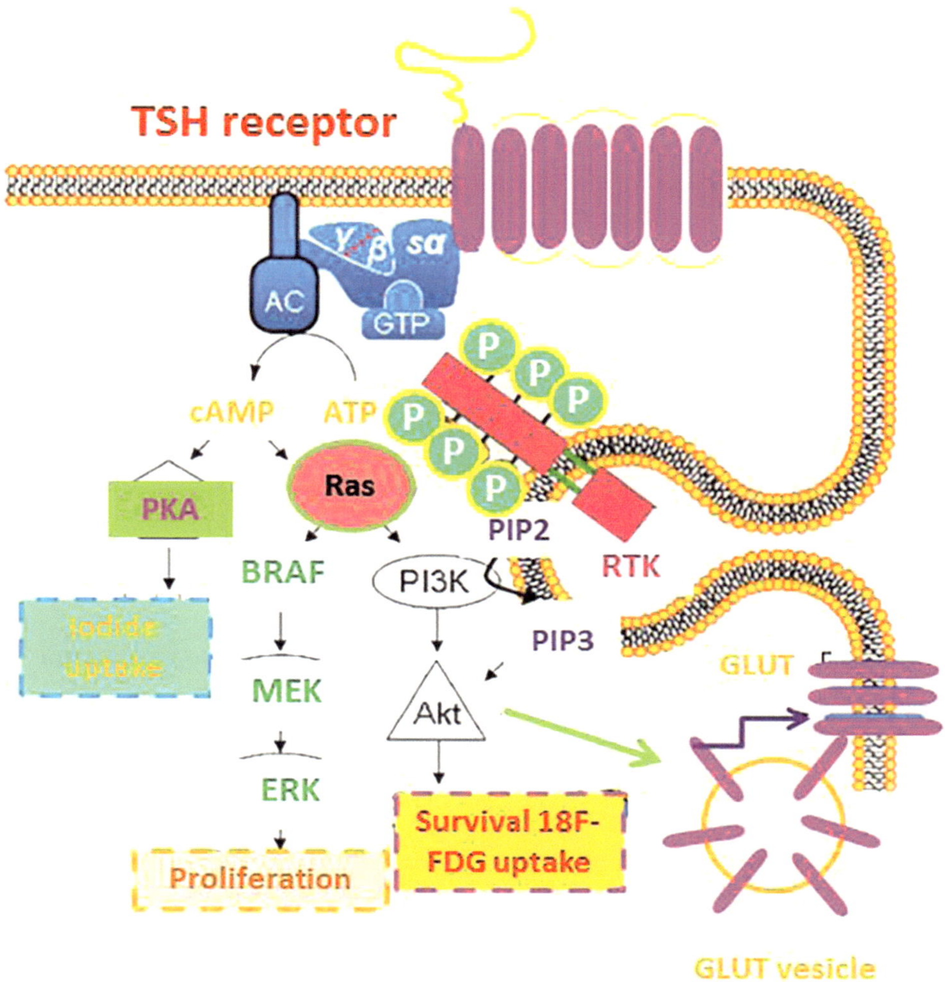

Figure 4.
According to Riesco-Eizaguirre and Santisteban, and Rivas and Santisteban, a proposed signal transduction pathway in the thyreocyte exist [36, 43]. The absorption of 18F-FDG triggered by TSH is mediated via adenylate cyclase (AC) and cAMP, as well as Ras, PI3K, and Akt. PKA regulates iodide absorption. The mitogen-activated protein (MAP) kinase pathway is hypothesized to control cell proliferation by involving B-type Raf (BRAF), extracellular signal-regulated kinase, and mitogen-activated protein kinase.

transfer of glucose, its catabolism to triose and pyruvate, and lastly to lactate. Due to the fact that glycolytic genes also respond directly to HIF-1, a collaboration between Myc and HIF has been seen in a number of cancers with genetic abnormalities [16, 120, 121]. In normoxia, Myc can accelerate glucose oxidation and lactate generation. Myc inhibits mitochondrial respiration with HIF-1 in order to create phosphoinositide-dependent kinase-1 and eventually favors anaerobic glycolysis (**Figure 5**) [122].

In addition to thyroid cancer, overexpression of c-Myc has been detected in a variety of other malignancies, where it promotes the expression of glucose metabolism genes. The c-Myc gene is a transcription factor that is associated with alterations in cellular metabolism and cancer. The initial connection between c-Myc and glycolysis was its influence on the positive regulation of an enzyme involved in the conversion of pyruvate from glycolysis to lactate. Additionally, c-Myc targets included glucose transporter-1, hexokinase 2, phosphofructokinase, and enolase 1 (**Figure 5**) [122].

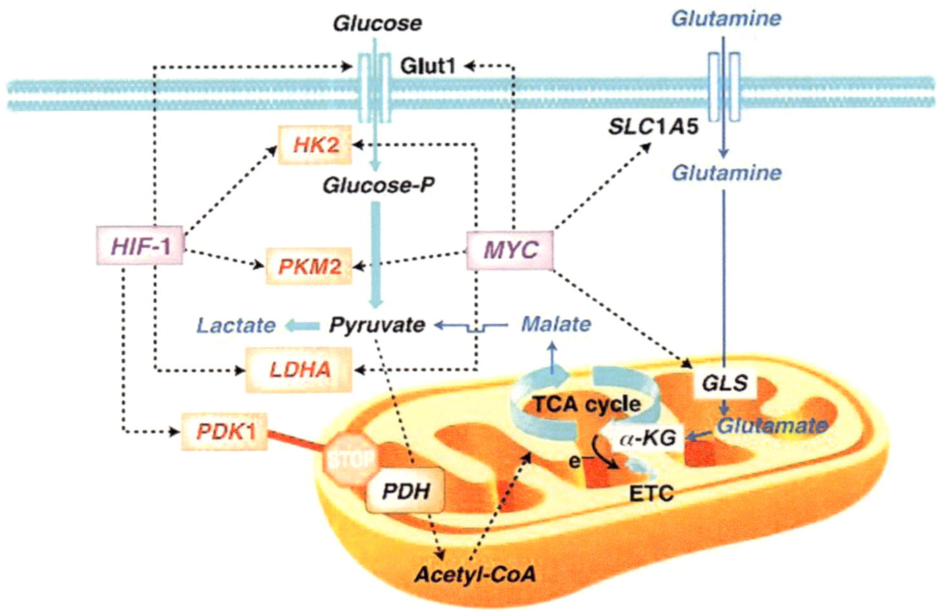

Figure 5.
Myc and HIF-1 are involved in the regulation of glucose metabolism and the Warburg effect. Myc and HIF-1 are shown to influence (dotted lines) glucose metabolism genes (glucose transporter Glut1, HK2, PKM2, LDHA, and PDK1), preferring glucose to lactate conversion (glycolysis). Myc is also shown to increase glutamine metabolism via the modulation of glutaminase and transporters (SLC1A5) (GLS).

4.5 AMPK

The reactive oxygen species (ROS) as upstream signals of AMP kinase (AMPK) can alter cellular metabolism and increase the Warburg effect by upregulation of AMPK. AMPK is a metabolic cytosolic enzyme that senses stress and is activated by a lack of energy for the regulation of metabolism and cell growth [123]. In contrast, ROS production is not controlled by AMPK. This is proven by inhibiting AMPK phosphorylation and evaluating ROS production under these conditions. AMPK plays an essential role in cell cycle arrest and has a strong anti-growth effect in various cancer cell lines.

In the thyroid gland, it plays a serious physiological role in the absorption of thyroid iodide in vitro and in vivo and can play a role in severe invasive thyroid cancer. When activated, AMPK promotes energy generation pathways and restores intracellular ATP levels, while simultaneously inhibiting energy consumption processes. AMPK activation also enhances glucose absorption in non-cancerous cells and papillary thyroid cancer cells, mostly in the first step of the glycolysis process. AMPK has been shown to increase glucose absorption in thyroid cells without requiring TSH by increasing both GLUT 1 expression and hexokinase (HK) activity.

This definitely suggests that AMPK regulates glucose absorption by thyrocytes via a different pathway. Two mechanisms that influence glucose metabolism include enhanced glucose transport to cells and increased glucose phosphorylation. Three kinases, including the liver kinase B1 homolog (serine/threonine protein kinase LKB1), calcium/calmodulin-dependent protein kinase kinase (CaMKK), and TGF-beta-activated kinase 1 (TAK1), may be involved in the control of thyrocyte glucose absorption. The capacity of AMPK to influence glucose metabolism may be valuable in discovering novel pathways involved in thyroid function regulation in the future [34, 124]. Inhibiting AMPK activation in tumor cells can enhance the Warburg effect. mTOR is significantly elevated in AMPK deficient models. Additionally, HIF-1 promotes the expression of HK2 and GLUT1, as well as glucose absorption by tumor cells. AMPK activation appears to contribute to the glucose metabolism seen in certain PTC cells. The active phosphorylated form of AMPK is expressed at a greater level in PTC tumor cell samples than in non-tumor tissue samples. Finally, more studies are necessary to clarify the role of AMPK in human thyroid cancer, particularly in metabolic regulation mechanisms such as cell proliferation, apoptosis, and survival [125–127].

5. Conclusion

While cancer was generally defined as aberrant cell growth, emerging data indicate that cancer is also a metabolic disorder. Metabolomics investigations, in addition to conventional approaches, are likely to be employed in the near future for the detection and classification of various forms of thyroid malignancies, most likely introducing altered metabolic pathways as treatment targets [128]. Thyroid cancer has a greater quick prevalence grade than any other kind of cancer in several countries [129]. Thyroid cancer cells have a high degree of metabolic complexity, indicating that they are capable of reprogramming glucose metabolism in response to nutritional restriction circumstances in the hypoxic tumor microenvironment. Malignant cells undergo metabolic alterations in order to get sufficient energy to continue growth signaling. Metabolic alterations such as increased glucose uptake are reported in invasive thyroid carcinoma for this purpose. Understanding the mechanisms of glucose transport to normal and pathological tissues of the thyroid can provide effective insights into the diagnosis and treatment of thyroid cancer treatments [27, 130].

Anticancer treatment is based on two main aspects. One is the traditional aspect of conventional chemotherapy, which is examined non-specifically against general cell processes. Another method is targeted molecular therapies, which include drugs designed to inhibit specific components of deregulated signaling pathways in cancer [131]. Deregulation of cellular metabolism as a hallmark of cancer may indicate changes in different signaling pathways. The metabolic change suggests a survival score for tumor cells [132]. Despite the number of various thyroid cancer biomarkers, only a few of them are clinically useful. Because one of these molecules may be ineffective on its own in many circumstances, the combination of two or more biomarkers can be quite helpful in detecting and predicting thyroid cancer [133]. The regulation of GLUTs is reviewed in this article in relation to critical amplification and survival pathways including as PI3K-Akt, HIF-1, MicroRNA, PTEN, AMPK, BRAF, c-Myc, and p53. Combination therapy is promising to enhance the efficacy of cancer treatment and cope with the multiple genetic alterations in different cancer cells. It involves simultaneous administration of more than one type of treatment such as two or more chemotherapies or merging chemotherapy with radiation/adjuvant therapy.

Because glucose uptake into cancer cells is a limiting step in glycolysis, nutritional restriction in tumors through targeting GLUTs by inhibiting their glucose transport channel with small molecules might be an acceptable approach [134]. Recently, the concept of cancer chemotherapy targeting glucose transporters has been highlighted [1]. Glucose transport inhibitors have been demonstrated to be potential anticancer medicines that need more investigation and clinical trials. As more information on cancer metabolism becomes available, we will be able to produce more effective anti-cancer treatments [39]. The discovery of the method of impaired glucose uptake through glucose-transporting proteins may alter the metabolism of malignant cells and thus disrupt tumor growth. If this hypothesis is confirmed, glucose-transporting proteins could become significant targets for cancer treatment [127]. Shifting the balance between cancer and stromal cells or the metabolic cooperation between different TC cell populations is a promising therapeutic strategy, but still needs further study. Finally, a better description of the metabolic phenotype under TC subtypes is clearly needed to provide a treatment option for poorly differentiated and refractory TC [130].

While conventional treatments such as surgical thyroidectomy and radioiodine therapy have been the main aspect of thyroid cancer treatment, they are frequently ineffective. As a result, treatment approaches against these sorts of malignancies must be recast in order to achieve modern drugs. Currently, the levels of GLUT1 or GLUT3 expression may give crucial information about the aggressiveness and growth of a tumor, as well as patient survival. The potential use of GLUTs as therapeutic targets is an exciting topic for future research in combination therapy.

Author details

Shabnam Heydarzadeh[1,2], Ali Asghar Moshtaghie[1], Maryam Daneshpour[2] and Mehdi Hedayati[2]*

1 Department of Biochemistry, School of Biological Sciences, Falavarjan Branch Islamic Azad University, Isfahan, Iran

2 Cellular and Molecular Endocrine Research Center, Research Institute for Endocrine Sciences, Shahid Beheshti University of Medical Sciences, Tehran, Iran

*Address all correspondence to: hedayati@endocrine.ac.ir

References

[1] Barron CC, Bilan PJ, Tsakiridis T, Tsiani E. Facilitative glucose transporters: Implications for cancer detection, prognosis and treatment. Metabolism. 2016;**65**:124-139

[2] Joost HG, Bell GI, Best JD, Birnbaum MJ, Charron MJ, Chen YT, et al. Nomenclature of the GLUT/SLC2A family of sugar/polyol transport facilitators. American Journal of Physiology. Endocrinology and Metabolism. 2002;**282**:974-976

[3] Szablewski L. Expression of glucose transporters in cancers. Biochimica et Biophysica Acta. 2013;**1835**:164-169

[4] Reinicke K, Sotomayor P, Cisterna P, Delgado C, Nualart F, Godoy A. Cellular distribution of Glut-1 and Glut-5 in benign and malignant human prostate tissue. Journal of Cellular Biochemistry. 2012;**113**:553-562

[5] Matsuzu K, Segade F, Matsuzu U, Carter A, Bowden DW, Perrier ND. Differential expression of glucose transporters in normal and pathological thyroid tissue. Thyroid. 2004;**14**:806-812

[6] Morani F, Pagano L, Prodam F, Aimaretti G, Isidoro C. Loss of expression of the oncosuppressor PTEN in associates with GLUT1 plasmamembrane expression. Panminerva Medica. 2012;**54**:59-63

[7] Younes M, Lechago LV, Lechago J. Overexpression of the human erythrocyte glucose transporter occurs as a late event in human colorectal carcinogenesis and is associated with an increased incidence of lymph node metastasis. Clinical Cancer Research. 1996;**2**:1151-1154

[8] Haber RS, Rathan A, Weiser KR, Pritsker A, Itzkowitz SH, Bodian C, et al. GLUT1 glucose transporter expression in colorectal carcinoma: A marker for poor prognosis. Cancer. 1998;**83**:34-40

[9] Koch A, Lang SA, Wild PJ, Gantner S, Mahli A, Spanier G, et al. Glucose transporter isoform 1 espression enhance metastasis of malignant melanoma cells. Oncotarget. 2015;**6**:32748-32760

[10] Amann T, Maegdefrau U, Hartmann A, Agaimy A, Marienhagen J, Weiss TS, et al. GLUT1 expression is increased in hepatocellular carcinoma and promotes tumorigenesis. The American Journal of Pathology. 2009;**174**:1544-1552

[11] Brown RS, Wahl RL. Overexpression of Glut-1 glucose transporter in human breast cancer, An immunohistochemical study. Cancer. 1993;**72**:2979-2985

[12] Ravazoula P, Batistatou A, Aletra C, Ladopoulos J, Kourounis G, Tzigounis B. Immunoisotchemical expression of glucose transporter Glut1 and cyclin D1 in breast carcinomas with negative lymph nodes. European Journal of Gynaecological Oncology. 2003;**24**:544-546

[13] Cantuaria G, Fagotti A, Ferrandina G, Magalhaes A, Nadji M, Angioli R, et al. GLUT-1 expression in ovarian carcinoma: Association with survival and response to chemotherapy. Cancer. 2001;**92**:1144-1150

[14] Semaan A, Munkarah AR, Arabi H, Bandyopadhyay S, Seward S, Kumar S, et al. Expression of GLUT-1 in epithelial ovarian carcinoma: correlation with tumor cell proliferation, angiogenesis, survival and ability to predict optimal cytoreduction. Gynecologic Oncology. 2011;**121**:181-186

[15] Coelho RG, Fortunato RS, Carvalho DP. Metabolic reprogramming in thyroid carcinoma, Thyroid Cancer

and Glycolysis. Frontiers in Oncology. 2018;**8**(82):1-15

[16] Dang CV, Kim JW, Gao P, Yustein J. The interplay between MYC and HIF in cancer. Nature Reviews. Cancer. 2008;**8**:51-56

[17] Bos R, van Der Hoeven JJ, van Der Wall E, van Der Groep P, van Diest PJ, Comans EF, et al. Biologic correlates of (18) fluorodeoxyglucose uptake in human breast cancer measured by positron emission tomography. Journal of Clinical Oncology. 2002;**20**:379-387

[18] Grabellus F, Nagarajah J, Bockisch A, Schmid KW, Sheu SY. Glucose transporter 1 expression, tumor proliferation, and iodine/glucose uptake in thyroid cancer with emphasis on poorly differentiated thyroid carcinoma. Clinical Nuclear Medicine. 2012;**37**:121-127

[19] Schönberger J, Rüschoff J, Grimm D, Marienhagen J, Rümmele P, Meyringer R, et al. Glucose transporter 1 gene expression is related to thyroid neoplasms with an unfavorable prognosis: An immunohistochemical study. Thyroid. 2002;**12**:747-754

[20] Bongiovanni M, Paone G, Ceriani L, Pusztaszeri M. Cellular and molecular basis for thyroid cancer imaging in nuclear medicine. Clinical and Translational Imaging. 2013;**1**:149-161

[21] Warburg O, Wind F, Negelein E. The metabolism of tumors in the body. Journal of General Physiology. 7 Mar 1927;**8**(6):519-530

[22] Warburg O. On the origin of cancer cells. Science. 1956;**123**:309-314

[23] Hatanaka M. Transport of sugars in tumor cell membranes. Biochimica et Biophysica Acta. 1974;**355**:77-104

[24] Isselbacher KJ. Sugar and amino acid transport by cells in culture—Differences between normal and malignant cells. The New England Journal of Medicine. 1972;**286**:929-933

[25] Isselbacher KJ. Increased uptake of amino acids and 2- deoxy-d-glucose by virus-transformed cells in culture. Proceedings of the National Academy of Sciences of the United States of America. 1972;**69**:585-589

[26] Suh HY, Choi H, Paeng JC, Cheon GJ, Chung JK, Kang KW. Comprehensive gene expression analysis for exploring the association between glucose metabolism and differentiation of thyroid cancer. BMC Cancer. 2019;**19**(1260):1-9

[27] Matsuzu K et al. Glucose transporters in the thyroid. Thyroid. 2005;**15**(6):545-550

[28] Schönberger J, Rüshoff J, Grimm D, Marienhagen J, Rümmele P, Meyringer R, et al. Glucose transporter 1 gene expression is related to thyroid neoplasms with an unfavorable prognosis: An immunohistochemical study. Thyroid. 2002;**12**:747-754

[29] Hooft L, van der Veldt AA, van Diest PJ, Hoekstra OS, Berkhof J, Teule GJ, et al. [18F]fluorodeoxyglucose uptake in recurrent thyroid cancer is related to hexokinase i expression in the primary tumor. The Journal of Clinical Endocrinology and Metabolism. 2005;**90**:328-334

[30] Yang H, Zhong J-T, Zhou S-H, Han H-M. Roles of GLUT-1 and HK-II expression in the biological behavior of head and neck cancer. Oncotarget. 2019;**10**(32):3066-3083

[31] Jozwiak P, Krzeslak A, Pomorski L, Lipinska A. Expression of hypoxia-related glucose transporters GLUT1 and GLUT3 in benign, malignant and non-neoplastic thyroid lesions. Molecular Medicine Reports. 2012;**6**:601-606

[32] Samih N, Hovsepian S, Aouani A, Lombardo D, Fayet G. Glut-1 translocation in FRTL-5 thyroid cells: role of phosphatidylinositol 3-kinase and N-glycosylation. Endocrinology. 2000;**141**:4146-4155

[33] Andrade BM, Cazarin J, Zancan P, Carvalho DP. AMP-activated protein kinase upregulates glucose uptake in thyroid PCCL3 cells independent of thyrotropin. Thyroid. 2012;**22**:1063-1068

[34] Bruno M. Andrade B. M., Cazarin J., and et al., AMP-activated protein kinase upregulates glucose uptake in thyroid PCCL3 cells independent of thyrotropin. Thyroid, 2012; 22(10): 1063-1068.

[35] Morani F, Pagano L, Prodam F, Aimaretti G, Isidoro C. Loss of expression of the oncosuppressor PTEN in thyroid incidentalomas associates with GLUT1 plasmamembrane expression. Panminerva Medica. 2012;**54**:59-63

[36] Xing M. Molecular pathogenesis and mechanisms of thyroid cancer. Nature Reviews. Cancer. 2013;**13**(3): 184-199

[37] Airley RE, Mobasheri A. Hypoxic regulation of glucose transport, anaerobic metabolism and angiogenesis in cancer: Novel pathways and targets for anticancer therapeutics. Chemotherapy. 2007;**53**:233-256

[38] Ganapathy V, Thangaraju M, Prasad PD. Nutrient transporters in cancer: Relevance to Warburg hypothesis and beyond. Pharmacology & Therapeutics. 2009;**121**:29-40

[39] Qian Y, Wang X, Chen X. Inhibitors of glucose transport and glycolysis as novel anticancer therapeutics. World Journal of Translational Medicine. 2014;**3**(2):37-57

[40] DeBerardinis RJ, Lum JJ, Hatzivassiliou G, Thompson CB. The biology of cancer: Metabolic reprogramming fuels cell growth and proliferation. Cell Metabolism. 2008;**7**:11-20

[41] Anastasiou D, Poulogiannis G, Asara JM, Boxer MB, Jiang JK, Shen M, et al. Inhibition of pyruvate kinase M2 by reactive oxygen species contributes to cellular antioxidant responses. Science. 2011;**334**:1278-1283

[42] Locasale JW, Grassian AR, Melman T, Lyssiotis CA, Mattaini KR, Bass AJ, et al. Phosphoglycerate dehydrogenase diverts glycolytic flux and contributes to oncogenesis. Nature Genetics. 2011;**43**:869-874

[43] Hsu PP, Sabatini DM. Cancer cell metabolism: Warburg and beyond. Cell. 2008;**134**:703-707

[44] Cairns RA, Harris IS, Mak TW. Regulation of cancer cell metabolism. Nature Reviews. Cancer. 2011;**11**:85-95

[45] Kroemer G, Pouyssegur J. Tumor cell metabolism: Cancer's Achilles' heel. Cancer Cell. 2008;**13**:472-482

[46] Garber K. Energy deregulation: licensing tumors to grow. Science. 2006;**312**:1158-1159

[47] Gatenby RA, Gillies RJ. Why do cancers have high aerobic glycolysis? Nature Reviews. Cancer. 2004;**4**:891-899

[48] Kim JW, Dang CV. Cancer's molecular sweet tooth and the Warburg effect. Cancer Research. 2006;**66**: 8927-8930

[49] Liu Y, Cao Y, Zhang W, Bergmeier S, Qian Y, Akbar H, et al. A smallmolecule inhibitor of glucose transporter 1 downregulates glycolysis, induces cell-cycle arrest, and inhibits cancer cell growth in vitro and in vivo. Molecular Cancer Therapeutics. 2012;**11**:1672-1682

[50] Ancey P-B, Contat C, Meylan E. Glucose transporters in cancer-from

tumor cells to the tumor microenvironment. The FEBS Journal. 2018;**285**:2926-2943

[51] Myers MP, Stolarov JP, Eng C, Li J, Wang SI, Wigler MH, et al. P-TEN, the tumor suppressor from human chromosome 10q23, is a dual-specificity phosphatase. Proceedings of the National Academy of Sciences of the United States of America. 1997;**94**: 9052-9057

[52] Phadngam S, Castiglioni A, Ferraresi A, Morani F, Follo C, Isidoro C. PTEN dephosphorylates AKT to prevent the expression of GLUT1 on plasmamembrane and to limit glucose consumption in cancer cells. Oncotarget. 2016;**7**(51):84999-85020

[53] Zarkesh M, Zadeh-Vakili A, Azizi F, Foroughi F, Akhavan MM, Hedayati M. Altered epigenetic mechanisms in thyroid cancer subtypes. Molecular Diagnosis & Therapy. 2018;**22**(1):41-56

[54] Razavi SA, Modarressi MH, Yaghmaei P, Tavangar SM, Hedayati M. Circulating levels of PTEN and KLLN in papillary thyroid carcinoma: Can they be considered as novel diagnostic biomarkers? Endocrine. 2017;**57**(3): 428-435

[55] Shinde SR, Maddika S. PTEN regulates glucose transporter recycling by impairing SNX27 retromer assembly. Cell Reports. 2017;**21**:1655-1666

[56] Morani F, Phadngam S, Follo C, Titone R, Aimaretti G, Galetto A, et al. PTEN regulates plasma membrane expression of glucose transporter 1and glucose uptake in thyroid cancer cells. Journal of Molecular Endocrinology. 2014;**53**(2):247-258

[57] Morani F, Phadngam S, Follo C, Titone R, Aimaretti G, Galetto A, et al. PTEN regulates plasma membrane expression of glucose transporter 1 and glucose uptake in thyroid cancer cells. Journal of Molecular Endocrinology. 2014;**53**:247-258

[58] Garcia-Cao I, Song MS, Hobbs RM, Laurent G, Giorgi C, de Boer VC, et al. Systemic elevation of PTEN induces a tumor-suppressive metabolic state. Cell. 2012;**149**:49-62

[59] Katoh H, Yamashita K, Enomoto T, Watanabe M. Classification and general considerations of thyroid cancer. Annals of Clinical Pathology. 2015;**3**(1):1045

[60] Zarkesh M, Zadeh-Vakili A, Akbarzadeh M, Fanaei SA, Hedayati M, Azizi F. The role of matrix metalloproteinase-9 as a prognostic biomarker in papillary thyroid cancer. BMC Cancer. 2018;**18**(1):1199

[61] Manzella L et al. New insights in thyroid cancer and P53 familly proteins. International Journal of Molecular Sciences. 2017;**18**(1325):1-15

[62] Quiros RM, Ding HG, Gattuso P, Prinz RA, Xu X. Evidence that one subset of anaplastic thyroid carcinomas are derived from papillary carcinomas due to BRAF and p53 mutations. Cancer. 2005;**103**:2261-2268

[63] Salvatore D, Celetti A, Fabien N, Paulin C, Martelli ML, Battaglia C, et al. Low frequency of p53 mutations in human thyroid tumours; p53 and Ras mutation in two out of fifty-six thyroid tumours. European Journal of Endocrinology. 1996;**134**:177-183

[64] Cancer Genome Atlas Research Network. Integrated genomic characterization of papillary thyroid carcinoma. Cell. 2014;**159**:676-690

[65] Dralle H, Machens A, Basa J, Fatourechi V, Franceschi S, Hay ID, et al. Follicular cell-derived thyroid cancer. Nature Reviews. Disease Primers. 2015;**1**:15077

[66] Garcia-Cao I, Song MS, Hobbs RM, et al. Systemic elevation of PTEN

induces a tumor-suppressive metabolic state. Cell. 2012;**149**:49-62

[67] Berkers CR, Maddocks OD, Cheung EC, Mor I, Vousden KH. Metabolic regulation by p53 family members. Cell Metabolism. 2013;**18**:617-633

[68] Maiuri MC, Galluzzi L, Morselli E, Kepp O, Malik SA, Kroemer G. Autophagy regulation by p53. Current Opinion in Cell Biology. 2010;**22**:181-185

[69] Muller PA, Caswell PT, Doyle B, et al. Mutant p53 drives invasion by promoting integrin recycling. Cell. 2009;**139**:1327-1341

[70] Morton JP, Timpson P, Karim SA, et al. Mutant p53 drives metastasis and overcomes growth arrest/senescence in pancreatic cancer. Proceedings of the National Academy of Sciences of the United States of America. 2010;**107**: 246-251

[71] Morani F, Phadngam S, Follo C, Titone R, Thongrakard V, Galetto A, et al. PTEN deficiency and mutant p53 confer glucose-addiction to thyroid cancer cells: impact of glucose depletion on cell proliferation, cell survival, autophagy and cell migration. Genes & Cancer. 2014;5(7-8):226-236

[72] Schwartzenberg-Bar-Yoseph F, Armoni M, Karnieli E. The tumor suppressor p53 down-regulates glucose transporters GLUT1 and GLUT4 gene expression. The American Journal of Cancer. Cancer Research. 2004;**64**: 2627-2633

[73] Bell GI, Kayano T, Buse JB, Burant CF, Takeda J, Lin D, et al. Molecular biology of mammalian glucose transporters. Diabetes Care. 1990;**13**:198-208

[74] Braun J, Hüttelmaier S. Pathogenic mechanisms of deregulated microRNA expression in thyroid carcinomas of follicular origin. Thyroid Research. 2011;**4**(1):S1

[75] Zhang B, Pan X, Cobb GP, Anderson TA. microRNAs as oncogenes and tumor suppressors. Developmental Biology. 2007;**302**:1-12

[76] Yue K, Wang X, Wu Y, Zhou X, He Q, Duan Y. microRNA-7 regulates cell growth, migration and invasion via direct targeting of PAK1 in thyroid cancer. Molecular Medicine Reports. 2016;**14**:2127-2134

[77] Ambros V. MicroRNA pathways in flies and worms: growth, death, fat, stress, and timing. Cell. 2003;**113**: 673-676

[78] Wang T, Xu H, Qi M, et al. miRNA dysregulation and the risk of metastasis and invasion in papillary thyroid cancer: A systematic review and meta-analysis. Oncotarget. 2018;**9**:5473-5479

[79] Perdas E, Stawski R, Nowak D, Zubrzycka M. Potential of liquid biopsy in papillary thyroid carcinoma in context of miRNA, BRAF and p53 mutation. Current Drug Targets. 1 Oct 2018;**19**(14):1721-1729

[80] Zarkesh M, Zadeh-Vakili A, Akbarzadeh M, Nozhat Z, Fanaei SA, Hedayati M, Azizi F. BRAF V600E mutation and microRNAs are helpful in distinguishing papillary thyroid malignant lesions: Tissues and fine needle aspiration cytology cases. Life Sciences. 15 Apr 2019;**223**:166-173

[81] Lien EC, Lyssiotis CA, Cantley LC. Metabolic Reprogramming by the PI3K-AktmTOR Pathway in Cancer. Recent Results in cancer Research Fortschritte der Krebsforschung Progres dans les recherches sur le Cancer. 2016;**207**:39-72

[82] Wang X, Qi M. miR-718 is involved in malignancy of papillary thyroid cancer through repression of PDPK1.

Pathology-Research and Practice. 1 Nov 2018;**214**(11):1787-1793

[83] Dettmer MS, Perren A, Moch H, Komminoth P, Nikiforov YE, Nikiforova MN. MicroRNA profile of poorly differentiated thyroid carcinomas: new diagnostic and prognostic insights. Journal of Molecular Endocrinology. 2014;**52**:181-189

[84] Huang P., Mao L., Zhang Z., Lv W., Feng X., Liao H., Dong CH., Kaluba B., Tang X., and Chang SH. Down-regulated miR-125a-5p promotes the reprogramming of glucose metabolism and cell malignancy by increasing levels of CD147 in thyroid cancer. Thyroid 2018; (0)0: 1-11.

[85] Filetti S, Vetri M, Damante G, Belfiore A. Thyroid autoregulation: Effect of iodine on glucose transport in cultured thyroid cells. Endocrinology. 1986;**118**(4):1395-1400

[86] Grabellus F, Nagarajah J, Bockisch A, Schmid K, Sien-Yi SS. Glucose Transporter 1 Expression, Tumor Proliferation, and Iodine/Glucose Uptake in Thyroid Cancer With Emphasis on Poorly Differentiated Thyroid Carcinoma. Clinical Nuclear Medicine. 2012;**37**(2):121-127

[87] Xing M. BRAF mutation in thyroid cancer. Endocrine-Related Cancer. 2005;**12**:245-262

[88] Nagarajah J et al. Correlation of BRAFV600E mutation and glucose metabolism in thyroid cancer patients: An 18F-FDG PET study. Journal of Nuclear Medicine. 2015;**56**(5):662-667

[89] Grabellus F et al. The BRAF V600E mutation in papillary thyroid carcinoma is associated with glucose transporter 1 overexpression. Thyroid. 2012;**22**(4):377-382

[90] Leonardi GC, Candido S, Carbone M, Raiti F, Colaianni V, Garozzo S, Cinà D, et al. BRAF mutations in papillary thyroid carcinoma and emerging targeted therapies. Molecular Medicine Reports. 1 Oct 2012;**6**(4):687-694

[91] Caronia LM, Phay JE, Shah MH. Role of BRAF in thyroid oncogenesis. Clinical Cancer Research. 2011;**17**(24):7511-7517

[92] Burrows N, Resch J, Cowen RL, Wasielewski R, Hoang-Vu C, West CM, et al. Expression of hypoxia-inducible factor 1α in thyroid carcinomas. Endocrine-Related Cancer. 2010;**17**:61-72

[93] Pouyssegur J, Dayan F, Mazure NM. Hypoxia signaling in cancer and approaches to enforce tumour regression. Nature. 2006;**441**:437-443

[94] Ciavardelli D, Bellomo M, Consalvo A, Crescimanno C, Vella V. Metabolic alterations of thyroid cancer as potential therapeutic targets. BioMed Research International. Oct 2017;**2017**:1-10

[95] Marin-Hernández A, Gallardo-Pèrez JC, Ralph SJ, Rodríguez-Enríquez S, Moreno-Sánchez R. HIF-1 alpha modulates energy metabolism in cancer by inducing over-expression of specific glycolytic isoforms. Mini Reviews in Medicinal Chemistry. 2009;**9**:1084-1101. DOI: 10.2174/138955709788922610

[96] Kalyanaraman B. Teaching the basics of cancer metabolism: Developing antitumor strategies by exploiting the differences between normal and cancer cell metabolism. Redox Biology. 2017;**12**:833-842

[97] Nozhat Z, Mohammadi-Yeganeh S, Azizi F, Zarkesh M, Hedayati M. Effects of metformin on the PI3K/AKT/FOXO1 pathway in anaplastic thyroid Cancer cell lines. Daru. 2018;**26**(2):93-103

[98] Klaus A, Fathi O, Tatjana TW, Bruno N, Oskar K. Expression of hypoxiaassociated protein HIF 1α in follicular thyroid cancer is associated with distant metastasis. Pathology Oncology Research. 2017;**2**:1-8

[99] Semenza GL. Targeting HIF-1 for cancer therapy. Nature Reviews. Cancer. 2003;**3**:721-732

[100] Denko NC. Hypoxia, HIF1 and glucose metabolism in the solid tumour. Nature Reviews Cancer. 2008;**8**:705-713

[101] Wong KK, Engelman JA, Cantley LC. Targeting the PI3K signaling pathway in cancer. Current Opinion in Genetics & Development. 2010;**20**:87-90

[102] Robbins H, Hague A. The PI3K/Akt pathway in tumors of endocrine tissues. Frontiers in Endocrinology. 2016;**6**(188):1-22

[103] Manning BD, Cantley LC. AKT/PKB signaling: Navigating downstream. Cell. 2007;**129**:1261-1274

[104] Barthel A, Okino ST, Liao J, Nakatani K, Li J, Whitlock JP Jr, et al. Regulation of GLUT1 gene transcription by the serine/threonine kinase Akt1. The Journal of Biological Chemistry. 1999;**274**:20281-20286

[105] Barron C, Bilan Ph, Tsakiridish, Tsiani E, Facilitative glucose transporters: Implications for cancer detection, prognosis and treatment. Metabolism, Clinical and Experimental 2016;65:124-139.

[106] Kroemer G, Pouyssegur J. Tumor cell metabolism: Cancer's Achilles heel. Cancer Cell. 2008;**13**:472-482

[107] Garcia-Rostan G, Zhao H, Camp RL, Pollan M, Herrero A, Pardo J, et al. Ras mutations are associated with aggressive tumor phenotypes and poor prognosis in thyroid cancer. Journal of Clinical Oncology. 2003;**21**(17):3226-3235

[108] Prante O, Maschauer S, Fremont V, Reinfelder J, Stoehr R, Szkudlinski M, et al. Regulation of uptake of 18F-FDG by a follicular human thyroid cancer cell line with mutation-activated K-Ras. Journal of Nuclear Medicine. 2009;**50**: 1364-1370

[109] Shaw RJ, Cantley LC. Ras, PI(3)K and mTOR signalling controls tumor cell growth. Nature. 2006;**441**:424-430

[110] Forbes SA, Beare D, Gunasekaren P, Leung K, Bindal N, Boutselakis H, et al. COSMIC: Exploring the world's knowledge of somatic mutations in human cancer. Nucleic Acids Research. 2015;**43**(21):805-811

[111] Nozhat Z, Hedayati M. PI3K/AKT pathway and its mediators in thyroid carcinomas. Molecular Diagnosis & Therapy. 2016;**20**(1):13-26

[112] Shan Jin S, Borkhuu O, Bao W, Yang Y. Signaling pathways in thyroid cancer and their therapeutic implications. Journal of Clinical Medical Research. 2016;**8**(4):284-296

[113] Chen M, Shen M, Li Y, et al. GC-MS-based metabolomics analysis of human papillary thyroid carcinoma tissue. International Journal of Molecular Medicine. 2015;**36**(6):1607-1614

[114] Moog F et al. Influence of thyroid-stimulating hormone levels on uptake of FDG in recurrent and metastatic differentiated thyroid carcinoma. The Journal of Nuclear Medicine. 2000;**41**(12):1989-1995

[115] Deichen JT, Schmidt C, Prante O, Maschauer S, Papadopoulos T, Kuwert T. Influence of TSH on uptake of [18F] fluorodeoxyglucose in human thyroid cells in vitro. European Journal of Nuclear Medicine and Molecular Imaging. 2004;**31**(4):507-512

[116] Brabant G, Maenhaut C, Kohrle J, Scheumann G, Dralle H, Hoang-Vu C,

et al. Human thyrotropin receptor gene: Expression in thyroid tumors and correlation to markers of thyroid differentiation and dedifferentiation. Molecular and Cellular Endocrinology. 1991;**82**:7-12

[117] Sabnis HS, Somasagara RR, Bunting KD. Targeting MYC dependence by metabolic inhibitors in cancer. Genes. 2017;**8**(114):1-20

[118] Kim JW, Gao P, Liu YC, Semenza GL, Dang CV. Hypoxia-inducible factor 1 and dysregulated c-Myc cooperatively induce vascular endothelial growth factor and metabolic switches hexokinase 2 and pyruvate dehydrogenase kinase 1. Molecular and Cellular Biology. 2007;**27**:7381-7393

[119] Kim JW, Zeller KI, Wang Y, et al. Evaluation of myc E-box phylogenetic footprints in glycolytic genes by chromatin immunoprecipitation assays. Molecular and Cellular Biology. 2004;**24**:5923-5936

[120] Dang CV, Le A, Gao P. MYC-induced cancer cell energy metabolism and therapeutic opportunities. Clinical Cancer Research. 2009;**15**(21):6479-6483

[121] Osthus RC, Shim H, Kim S, et al. Deregulation of glucose transporter 1 and glycolytic gene expression by c-Myc. The Journal of Biological Chemistry. 2000;**275**:21797-21800

[122] Ohta K, Endo T, Onaya T. The mRNA levels of thyrotropin receptor, thyroglobulin and thyroid peroxidase in neoplastic human thyroid tissues. Biochemical and Biophysical Research Communications. 1991;**174**:1148-1153

[123] Wu CA, Chao Y, Shiah SG, Lin WW. Nutrient deprivation induces the Warburg effect through ROS/AMPK-dependent activation of pyruvate dehydrogenase kinase. Biochimica et Biophysica Acta. 2013;**1833**:1147-1156

[124] Cazarin JM, Coelho RG, Hecht F, Andrade BM, Carvalho DP. 5'-AMPactivated protein kinase regulates papillary (TPC1 and BCPAP) thyroid cancer cell survival, migration, invasion and epithelial-to-mesenchymal transition. Thyroid. 2016;**26**:933-942

[125] Luo Z, Zang M, Guo W. AMPK as a metabolic tumor suppressor: Control of metabolism and cell growth. Future Oncology. 2010;**6**:457-470

[126] Faubert B, Boily G, Izreig S, Griss T, Samborska B, Dong Z, et al. AMPK is a negative regulator of the Warburg effect and suppresses tumor growth in vivo. Cell Metabolism. 2013;**17**:113-124

[127] Vidal AP, Andrade BM, Vaisman F, Cazarin J, Pinto LF, Breitenbach MM, et al. AMP-activated protein kinase signaling is upregulated in papillary thyroid cancer. European Journal of Endocrinology. 2013;**169**:521-528

[128] Nozhat Z, Hedayati M, Azizi F. Thyroid Cancer Epidemic: A Peril or an Alarm?. International Journal of Endocrinology and Metabolism. Oct 2015;**13**(4):1-2

[129] Nozhat Z, Hedayati M, Azizi F. Thyroid cancer epidemic: A peril or an alarm? International Journal of Endocrinology and Metabolism. 2015;**13**(4)

[130] Burrows N, Resch J, Cowen RL, Von Wasielewski R, Hoang-Vu C, West CM, et al. Expression of hypoxia-inducible factor 1α in thyroid carcinomas. Endocrine-related Cancer. Mar 2010;**17**(1):61

[131] Macheda ML, Rogers S, Best JD. Molecular and cellular regulation of glucose transporter (GLUT) proteins in cancer. Journal of Cellular Physiology. 2005;**202**:654-662

[132] Calvo MB, Figueroa A, Pulido EG, Campelo RG, Aparicio LA. Potential

role of sugar transporters in cancer and their relationship with anticancer therapy. International Journal of Endocrinology. Oct 2010;**2010**:1-14

[133] Nozhat Z, Azizi F, Hedayati M. A review on molecular biomarkers of thyroid carcinoma. Journal of Mazandaran University of Medical Sciences. 2015;**25**(125):154-170

[134] Granchi C, Fancelli D, Minutolo F. An update on therapeutic opportunities offered by cancer glycolytic metabolism. Bioorganic & Medicinal Chemistry Letters. 2014;**24**:4915-4925